LAMENESS

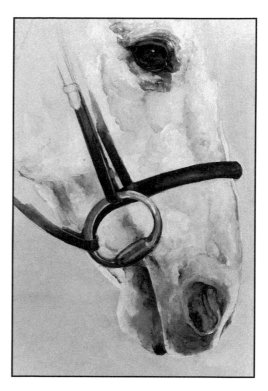

LAMENESS

Peter Gray
MVB, MRCVS

J. A. Allen
London

To Sean, Michael, Paul and Allin

British Library Cataloguing in Publication Data
A catalogue record for this book is available from the British Library

ISBN 0 85131 577 1

Published in Great Britain in 1994 by
J. A. Allen & Company Limited
1 Lower Grosvenor Place
London SW1W 0EL

Production editor: Bill Ireson
Illustrator: Maggie Raynor
Series designer: Nancy Lawrence
Printed in Great Britain by The Bath Press, Avon

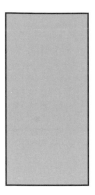

Contents

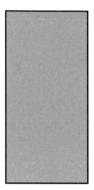

Introduction

The purpose of writing a book on lameness is to create a greater awareness of the subject and to present to everyone who rides or keeps horses the idea of the prevention of lameness. We who are in daily contact with horses are privileged, despite the drudgery involved and the material demands of a cost-consuming luxury. The prevention of lameness is, therefore, owed to the animal, but we also benefit from the potential elimination of the cost of treatment, or even the mere loss of use.

Prevention of lameness is not a new subject, but one broached repeatedly. It may well start with good shoeing and dedicated supervision of foot care, but it proceeds through understanding of conformation and anatomy, appreciation of the demands of physical development, the influence of concussion, and the working of systems such as the muscles, bones and particularly the spinal skeleton.

All of these aspects are highlighted in this book and it is my hope that they will become more widely understood. If that happens, the horse will also benefit and the whole exercise will have been worthwhile.

The basis of lameness prevention is as follows:

1)   Foot and limb balance are essential to the prevention of sprains, strains and conditions such as angular deformity. Shoeing is an essential element of this.

2)   The correct approach to concussion absorption can prevent the development of ringbone, sidebone, splints and spavin.

3)   Constitutional lamenesses are prevented by proper feeding and an understanding of diet management (e.g. over-feeding of young animals may lead to osteochondritis; improper diet management can lead to azoturia).

4)   Understanding the muscular system is a means of preventing not only muscular lameness but also secondary lameness resulting from it. It is also a significant factor in tendon injuries and is closely allied to lameness of spinal origin.

5)   Early diagnosis and proper care of spinal origin lameness is best achieved on a regular preventive basis, especially in known sufferers.

6)   Good shoeing is a basis for preventing a whole range of common modern lamenesses.

Approaching equine lameness from the viewpoint of cause and effect is a move away from the standard approach, which has been almost universally based on the hypothesis that the vast majority of lameness occurs in the areas from the knee to the ground in the forelimb and from the hock to the ground in the hind limb. Modern clinical experience, objectively assessed, has to take us to a wider understanding of the problem particularly as it affects the athletic animal. While no statistics are available to refute the old idea, there is adequate living proof that other sources of lameness (e.g. the muscular system and the skeleton) are all now common enough today to challenge that status.

Under the Veterinary Surgery (Exemptions) Order 1962, treatment of an animal by physiotherapy is permitted by a non-veterinarian as long as the animal has first been examined by a vet who referred it for such treatment. Physiotherapy, in this context, is taken to include all forms of manipulative therapy and there are no stipulations as to the qualifications to be held by such therapists. That there are is not good enough and it leaves the door open to all forms of clinical abuse; many people who attend horses unsupervised under the guise of 'physiotherapist' are without a basic understanding of the subject. Animals are made to suffer through human exploitation, and the situation demands redress.

Peter Gray

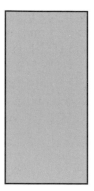

Acknowledgements

My thanks to the following: David Watson, BA, MRCVS, for reading and editing the manuscript; Brendan Paterson, BVetMed CertESM, MRCVS, for his help with the manuscript and for providing radiographswhich have been used in this book; Mrs D. A. Sinclair LLB, Assistant Registrar of the Royal College of Veterinary Surgeons for advice relating to the introduction.

I have acknowledged sources for illustrations in the individual captions throughout the book; for permission to reproduce material I am grateful to the following individuals and institutions: John Birt; Victory Racing Company, Baltimore, USA and their British agent, Atlantic Equine Limited, Rugby, England; Mustad Hoofcare SA, Switzerland and their British agent, EPC of Frome, Somerset, England; G. Stonehewer of Universal Horse Shoes, Ludlow, England; Sue Devereux, BVSc, MRCVS; L. Rochford, MCSP; and Stuart Newsham.

My special thanks to Maggie Raynor, for her excellent artwork, to Bill Ireson, for his production editing, and to my publishers.

Author Note
I have used everyday and common terms when naming parts of the horse. In veterinary practice, of course, technical names are used for greater accuracyof definition. Where it will aid the reader, therefore, I have occasionally used both in the text.

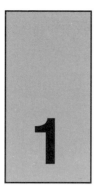

Causes of Lameness

Lameness may result from any of a number of factors, though some have a more persistent influence than others. For example:

1)   Concussion (now termed axial compression force) plays a complex part in a high percentage of lameness conditions. It is best understood as the force which is transmitted to the limb each time a horse's foot strikes the ground. Body weight also acts down through the limb at the point of ground contact and may instigate lameness if the bulk of its influence has to be disproportionately received by any single part.

2)   Movement is basic to the previous influences because a stationary animal is not exposed to concussion, and body weight alone is unlikely to lead to lameness on the same basis (with the exception of an already lame animal having to bear too much weight on a single limb).

3)   Conformation decides to a certain extent, how each limb deals with the axial forces it is subjected to.

4)   Terrain also has an important influence on lameness, depending on whether ground is hard or soft, uneven, pot-holed or false (alternating hard and soft).

5)   Trauma is the inadvertent injury of anatomical structures. The only solution to trauma is prevention by having safe fences, good working surfaces, etc. However, there is still the physical nature of the animal to contend with.

6)   Infection occurs most commonly as a result of natural (grit, splinters, thorns) or human (shoeing) intrusions.

7)   Nutrition is a factor in lameness, largely due to the development and growth of cartilage and bone. It can also be a precipitating factor in conditions affecting the muscular system.

8)   Foot balance and shoeing are critical factors because of the fundamental relationship that exists between these and axial forces.

Important Anatomical Points of the Horse

1)   The head, for purely descriptive purposes, is defined as a heavy bob-weight suspended at the end of a long, adjustable lever, the neck. This arrangement, rotating from the front of a virtually fixed trunk, permits the horse to alter its centre of gravity, or balance, at will. Furthermore, while the head and neck play no direct part in progression, they give attachment to muscles originating in the forelimb and trunk that are critically involved in forelimb movement. Lameness associated with the head and neck is caused by muscular injuries as well as that which has its origin in spinal structures.

2)   The forelimb is attached to the body by muscle and ligament only. There is no bony attachment of forelimb to the spine; there being no clavicle in the equine. This influences movement and also the manner in which concussion is absorbed by the limb. While the forelimbs are employed mainly to receive weight, they also have an important part to

The centre of gravity varies with body position: as the horse's head is lowered the centre of gravity moves forward and down

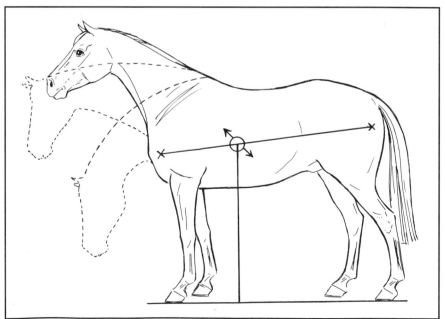

play in moving off and propulsion. However, in a standing animal, 60 per cent of the body weight is carried by the forelimbs and this ultimately influences the incidence of lameness. The front limbs bear the main brunt of concussion experienced in movement, because it is they that take the weight of a horse coming down from a jump. This is reflected in the higher incidence of concussive lameness in these limbs, e.g. pedal osteitis, ringbone, sesamoiditis, splints, sore shins, carpitis, etc. Navicular disease also has a concussive element to it in many cases.

3)   How these forces are received is influenced by anatomical construction and by the particular conformational attributes of individual animals.

a) The knee (or carpus), being inserted in a straight line between the radius and metacarpal bones, has no option but to meet the forces it is subjected to in a very direct manner. Furthermore, the degree of movement in individual knee joints means that their position at the point of ground contact often brings a natural backward influence on the bones.

The conformation of the knee is therefore critical to its soundness and its ultimate ability to withstand the normal forces it is subjected to.

The forearm, knee and cannon are normally held in a straight line as the limb bears weight

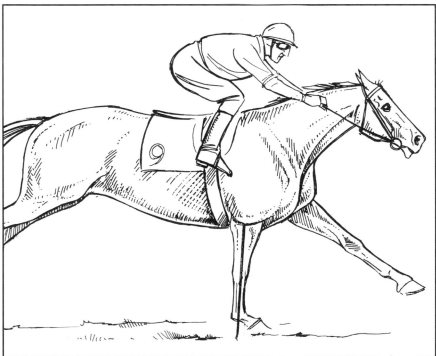

b) The fetlock, being set at an angle of 145 degrees to the pastern, is supported at its rear by the superficial and deep flexor tendons, the suspensory apparatus and the annular ligament of the joint itself. It is a joint that has a great deal of movement, and one of its functions is to direct axial forces directly up or down the limb without endangering its own integrity. Failure to achieve this results in injuries to any of the structures involved.

c) The pastern, being supported behind by tendons and ligaments, is also relatively shielded from direct trauma. It is most commonly challenged in immature animals when bone is not fully strengthened. It is at its weakest in long limbed young animals.

d) The foot and pastern are set in such a way that, ideally, a line drawn along the front surface of each breaks neither backwards or forwards. The foot being a complex structure has its own in-built anti-concussive parts.

Structures supporting the fetlock joint

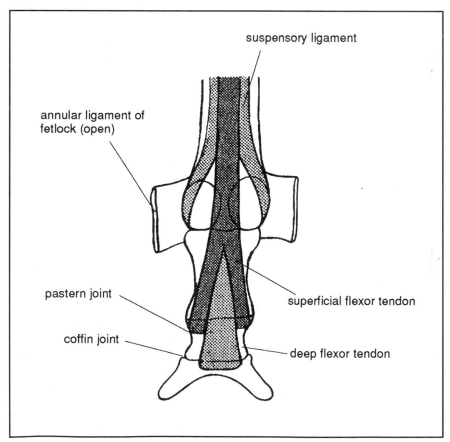

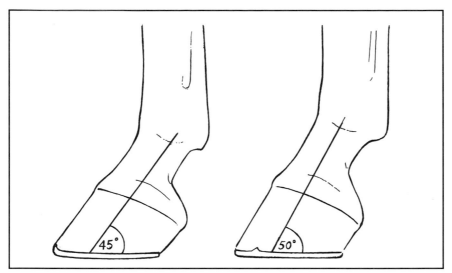

Normal foot/pastern angle in fore and hind limb

However, any break from normal in the foot/pastern axis is likely to lead to lameness as a result of the stresses this creates. The normal foot/pastern axis is 45 degrees for the forelimb and 50 degrees for the hind limb.

4)   The hind limb, the power house of locomotion, forms a bony attachment to the pelvis through the hip joint. The pelvis in turn is attached to the sacrum through the sacroiliac joint, a form of ligamentous attachment that is a modified true synovial joint. Concussion is therefore transmitted through the pelvis directly to the spinal column, and is partly absorbed by the intervertebral discs, especially in the lumbar region.

5)   The horse gallops by generating most of its hind limb advancement through the stifle and hock joints. It also flexes its spine, though the extent of this is strictly limited. One of the most important joints in the locomotory system, the hock, also plays an important part in the absorption of concussion.

Stifle and hock work in coordination, not individually. This double function is operated by means of two opposing sets of muscles, known as the reciprocal mechanism. It means a great deal of concussion in the hind limb is counteracted by means of combined hock and stifle flexion. The hock combines two kinds of joint: one is capable of free undirectional movement - a ginglymus (hinge) joint; the other is only involved in more direct shock absorption - arthrodial (gliding) joints.

6)   The stifle is a compound joint incorporating union between the femur and tibia on the one hand and that between the femur and patella on the other. The joint surfaces communicate through the synovial capsules

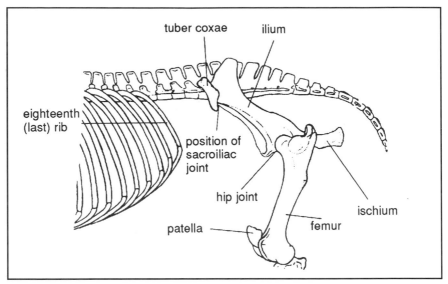

Attachment of the hind limb to the pelvis at the hip and to the spine at the sacroiliac joint

and work together in cooperation. The stifle's significance in concussion absorption is important, especially because it distributes this effect to the large muscle masses attached to it and, through the femur, to the pelvis, spine and body.

7)   The vertebral column has limited flexibility in the thoracic and lumbar regions and effectively none in the sacrum. It is capable of only minor movement dorsoventrally and laterally. The extent of this has been estimated to be limited to 10-12cm laterally in a supple horse. To achieve acute turns in confined spaces, the horse pivots on its hind feet and abducts its limbs.

The incidence of spinal-origin lameness is an extremely significant factor in ridden horses. While, fortunately, not many injuries sustained are of a permanent nature, a large number cause impaired movement and lameness. In many of these cases manipulation and physiotherapy are the rational answer.

This problem is not experienced in any other animal to the same extent and we should therefore be aware of the nature of the equine spine and what we are entitled to ask of it.

8)   The movement that does occur in the thoracolumbar region is found between individual thoracic vertebrae, between the last thoracic and first lumbar, between the first three lumbar, and at the lumbosacral junction. This movement is necessarily dependent to a great extent upon the

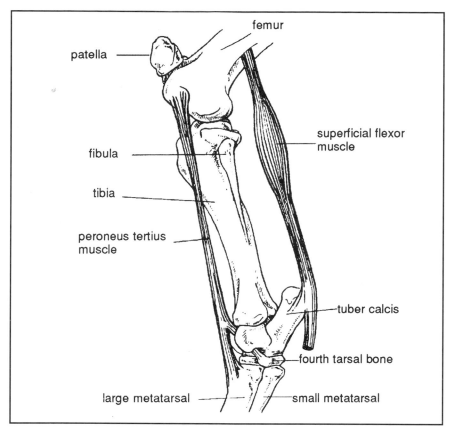

Reciprocal apparatus of the hind limb

thickness of the intervertebral discs, which are firmly united to the bodies of the vertebrae. With advanced years calcification is common and further outgrowths of bone may act as bridges between bones making union almost complete.

In the synovial articulations between the transverse processes of one or more of the last three lumbar vertebrae, an active arthritis may occur as early as the second or third year, resulting in solid fusion (spondylosis), often with the formation of fresh bony deposits surrounding the actual joints. This process (known as ankylosis) does not normally include the lumbosacral joint. It means there can be no further movement in the affected joint.

9)   The vertebral column, being the axis upon which the limbs act to produce movement, is flexed in the thoracolumbar area by forces produced by the thrust of the hind limbs against the ground. Both oblique and vertical forces are exerted on the spine by the hind limbs. Oblique forces

are exhibited as a tendency to flex the spine sideways, while vertical forces tend to increase the curvature of the thoracolumbar bow, i.e. to flex it vertically. Sideways forces and the resultant lateral oscillation are clearly apparent at the walk. At speeds higher than that, however, muscular resistance makes the column as rigid as possible in order to eliminate sideways movement.

Above the spinal column the *longissimus dorsi* muscle and below it the *psoas minor* cooperate by simultaneous contraction in an effort to counter attempts at flexion. When the synchronisation between these muscles fails, as during a fall or even galloping on level ground - and sometimes during recovery from anaesthesia - fracture of the back may occur. The damage usually takes place in the thoracic region.

10)   The pelvic roof is an area subject to the direct mechanical forces of hind limb action. The result is that muscular injuries are common on the upper part of the quarter and in the large muscle masses running down to the stifle. Minor displacements of the sacrum in relation to the ilium result in sacroiliac joint disease which is not an uncommon occurrence. It

Points in movement which may adversely influence spinal anatomy

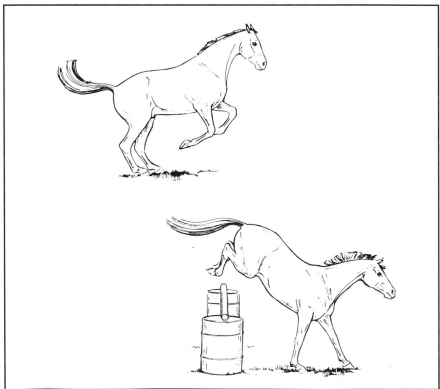

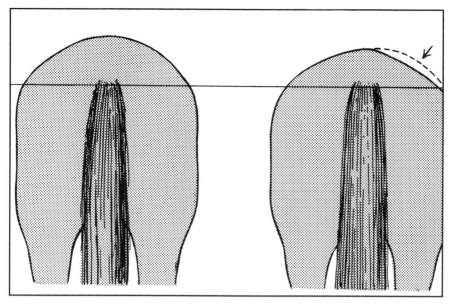

Atrophy of muscle here (arrowed) *may result from sacroiliac injuries or from primary muscular injuries*

is also not unknown for the tail to be broken and any abnormality in its use may indicate more serious disruption of spinal function.

11)   The health of the horse's muscular system is of great importance. Its significance is often ignored, because, when injured, it only produces lameness that lasts for a limited period. Within a matter of days of initial injury, the animal returns to a relative degree of soundness, and an accompanying alteration of gait is either not seen or disregarded. Yet the importance of this alteration is significant because it not only impedes movement but also commonly leads to secondary lameness, which may often be expressed by tendon ruptures, or injury to more rigid structures of the limbs.

Axial Forces

Concussion takes effect at the moment weight is borne (inevitably increasing with pace). However, it is not only the direct influence of upward jarring that affects each anatomical structure but also the downward influence of body weight pressing from above. As already stated, the individual anatomy (and conformation) of each limb joint has a bearing on how this is received: the angulation and manner in which bones meet

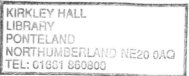

The way weight is borne is affected by conformation. The effect of body weight downwards is of great importance, as is the influence of ground forces upwards

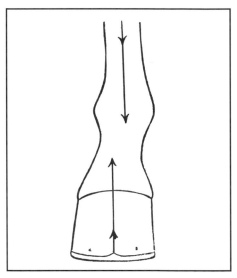

being critical to the kind of stress that is suffered. Any weakness will eventually decide the limb's ability to deal with these varying forces.

The ultimate influence, then, is the way in which natural anatomy meets everyday stresses of locomotion. A joint, ligament or tendon which is subjected to abnormal loading because of intrinsic faulty limb design, or resulting from an extrinsic cause (such as improper shoeing, or placing a limb in a hole), is more likely to be injured. This particularly applies to the young, strongly growing animal when the development of deformity at joints such as the knee or fetlock may result from lack of foot care, and/or immaturity. The same often applies to splints that suddenly appear in older horses. It is loss of limb balance that is expressed as specific lameness, not the reverse.

The equine limb was designed with an ideal in mind: to protect individual sectors from being subjected to disproportionate strain. That there is lameness is an indication that this ideal is not always met, and that our understanding, at times, fails to protect the underlying aim.

Other Influences

Lameness, of course, also occurs unavoidably. Trauma is a natural consequence of physical activities that sometimes defy nature. The horse was not designed for its ability to jump and, therefore, the act of jumping poses problems for the structures of the vertebral column. Our failure to consider the basic demands of a healthy muscular system also causes injuries which, often, are avoidable, and the consequence of which is frequently more serious lameness.

Even when conformation is ideal, there is never any way of fully preventing the possibility of a horse meeting a hole when travelling at speed. Tendon injuries also may occur as a result of a limb being overstretched mechanically, as when landing awkardly after a jump. But these injuries can also be the legacy of faulty training techniques, of too much hurry in getting animals fit, or of selecting bad ground to exercise on, and they may appear as secondary conditions when other mechanical limitations on movement - such as muscle damage - place an undue strain on any single structure.

What all this means is that a certain amount of lameness can be prevented; a certain amount cannot.

However, if our understanding of the causes was more widely considered, the total wastage due to this perennial problem would be markedly reduced.

Concussion is met by the limb and body as described in the following sequence:

1)   The foot - in particular the frog, digital cushion, cartilages, etc. - allows for a certain amount of absorption and is designed in such a way as to limit the effect on each individual structure involved.

2)   The backward inclination of the pastern and its tendoligamentous supports assists this.

3)   The construction of the fetlock and sesamoids with the strong lig-

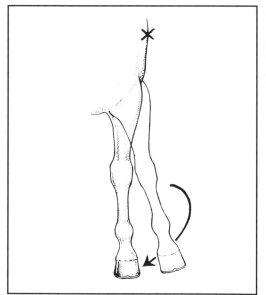

Muscular injury can alter limb action: the site of the injury (X) can alter the outward movement (arrowed) of the limb due to the shortening of muscle in the injured area

amentous bonding and tendinous support helps save these structures and steer axial forces up through the cannon.

4)   The knee and hock act as shock absorbers.

5)   The angulation of the elbow/shoulder joints in front and the hock/stifle/hip joints behind play their part as well.

6)   The muscle masses of the upper limb absorb concussion.

7)   Finally, the trunk and spine are affected.

It is evident that any weakness on this anatomical line can lead to injury in the region where the weakness exists.

Thus, if the frontal angulation of the limb when it meets the ground is away from the perpendicular, the site where weakness exposes itself may be where a perpendicular line from the centrepoint of ground contact emerges through either aspect of the limb. The result may be sprain, strain or fracture of any of the structures involved. However, the downward influence of body weight also has a bearing here.

The Forelimb

The natural construction of the forelimb conducts axial forces in a straight line, making sure that their influence is absorbed in a manner that effects least stress to any one anatomical part.

Take a frontal view of the limb in a weight-bearing position. The foot should bear evenly on either side of the midline so that there is no inclination for the inner and outer walls to be disproportionate, thus placing the foot (and limb) out of balance.

This design affords the limb maximum strength in a weight-bearing position and so limits the loading of individual features. No defect, deformity or interference should cause the central bisecting line to break either inwardly or outwardly from the point of ground contact upwards.

The frontal line through the pastern should bisect the fetlock, cannon, knee and forearm (when continued upwardly). This enables the limb to act as a strut on ground contact, in a way that ensures maximum strength and allows the opposing forces of concussion and body weight to meet in a way that avoids injury, including fracture.

The effect of concussion is thereafter absorbed through the elbow and shoulder into the muscle masses of the upper body and trunk, and indirectly to the spine; the influence of body weight moving downwards is received with minimal risk of injury. (The fact that the scapula is curved onto the body does not alter this principle.)

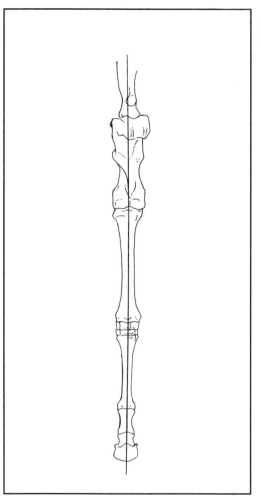

Ideally, axial forces are absorbed in a straight line as weight is borne

It is critical that the foot be balanced and meets the ground at an angle between 45 and 50 degrees in profile, as already mentioned; an angle that will be roughly parallel to a line drawn along the spine of the scapula. Thus an upright pastern will very often be associated with a straight shoulder (though the shoulder angle may be dictated by the relative lengths of the scapula and humerus).

The angle of the front of the foot should carry through the front of the pastern without breaking backward or forward. If the heels are too low and the toe too long, it breaks backward and this type of conformation can place unwanted strain on the structures at the back of the limb, including the navicular bone, tendons and suspensory ligament. It can also affect the bones of the knee.

Improper foot balance can affect higher limb structures

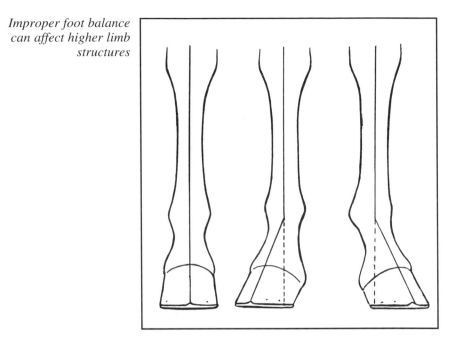

If the foot is too upright and the heels too high, the line is broken forward and this can cause contraction of the frog in some instances and increase concussion to vital limb structures like the fetlock and cannon bone.

In certain cases, foot balance may be disturbed because of inherent faulty conformation elsewhere. Deviations at fetlock or knee may cause

Long toe/low heel (left) *affects the lower limb joints and places a strain on the flexor tendons. Short toe/high heel conformation* (right) *increases pressure on the fetlock and coffin joints*

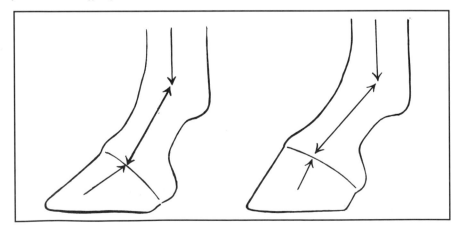

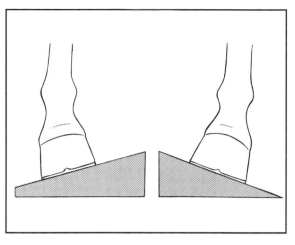

Uneven ground (which can include road camber) may cause full body weight to be borne abnormally by limb joints

the bearing angle of a well-balanced foot to be unlevel. The consequent effect may mean that concussion is absorbed mainly by the faulty joint (or lower structures affected by it), thereby having serious limitations on the animal's ability to remain sound.

As happens with human athletes, it is vital that this imbalance be altered - in horses, by corrective shoeing, when possible, even if this means the animal spending its life wearing shoes which are different in thickness between outer and inner branches. The important thing is that the animal be protected from the effects of its own, perhaps slight, anatomical divergence. The result can often be an extension of useful, natural life.

In order to elaborate on this we shall treat the foot, fetlock, knee and forearm separately, taking conformational faults as a basis of discussion in each case.

The Foot and Pastern

Foot balance is critical to total leg balance and it is sometimes necessary to alter what appear to be natural foot levels in order to avoid injury to other limb structures.

The ultimate criterion of good shoeing is the way the foot strikes the ground. The foot level must be correct, otherwise a level shoe will not meet the ground on a level plane. For this reason it is necessary that a horse be walked and trotted for the farrier before shoeing, so that the shape and action can be gauged and the foot trimmed accordingly, making sure it is fully balanced. It is also imperative that the finished shoe itself be level, otherwise the whole balance of the limb is disturbed.

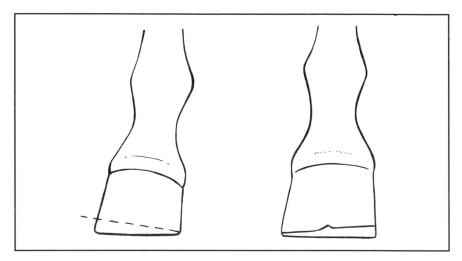

Abnormal foot balance is corrected by trimming or, where this is not feasible, by altering the level of the shoe

Certain types of shoe, for example, contain areas for providing grip on slippery surfaces; it is not uncommon for these to wear unevenly, thus leaving a shoe which is unsuitable at ground surface. Not only is it unsuitable, but it loses stability and 'rocks'. The result can easily be injury to joints indirectly influenced by this.

Following the plane of the bearing surface, note how a shortening of the wall either medially or laterally upsets the whole balance of the limb

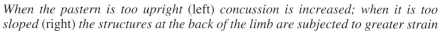

When the pastern is too upright (left) *concussion is increased; when it is too sloped* (right) *the structures at the back of the limb are subjected to greater strain*

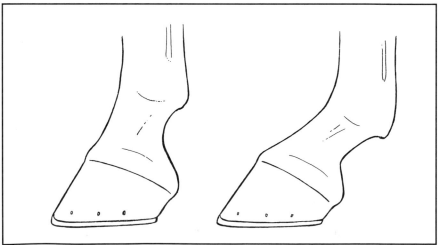

in relation to the ground and influences the path of concussive forces travelling upwards. These imbalances also affect forces coming down the limb - due to body weight. Lameness commonly results, and is almost inevitable eventually if the fault is not corrected. Also visualise how elongation of the toe, lowering of the heel and dumping (shortening the toe by rasping the outside wall) of the front of the foot all affect the foot/pastern axis and influence soundness in a similar way.

It is the purpose of the shoe to protect the foot from undue wear, to limit concussion, and to spread its effect through the structures of the foot in a natural way. To achieve this, the frog, digital cushion, cartilages, and blood plexuses must all function normally. In addition, there must be no pressure on sensitive tissues, and no bruising from nail or shoe on structures which may become inflamed or infected.

The Fetlock

The fetlock comes under abnormal stress when the limb axis is out of line. This joint bears a large percentage of axial forces in motion, but especially when a horse is landing from a jump. At this point, any weakness can lead to serious injury; good management should ensure that this does not happen because of avoidable problems, like improper limb balance or the choice of unsuitable ground.

The Knee

The knee is largely protected from the influence of axial forces by its anatomical position between the radius and large metacarpal bones. However, this protection is compromised by conformation that tends to be back-at-the-knee; and also by fatigue (most typically at the end of a race) when the fetlock in a weight-bearing position falls lower to the ground and the straight alignment of the radius/carpus/metacarpus is consequently broken backwards.

This straight alignment is also lost from an anteroposterior (front to back) viewpoint in angular deformities which result in abnormal development of the growth plates, especially of the radius, and in bench-knee conformation.

Surface Influences

Concussion is influenced by camber, surface and the increasing hardness

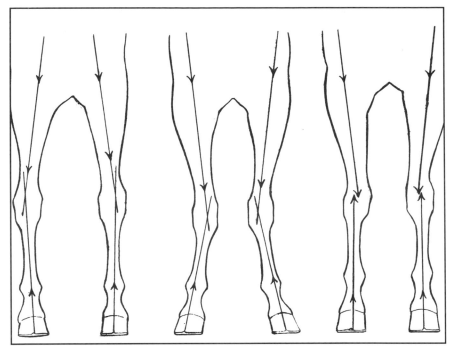

Knee conformation is critical to soundness

These bench knees did not predispose to lameness in this ridden horse

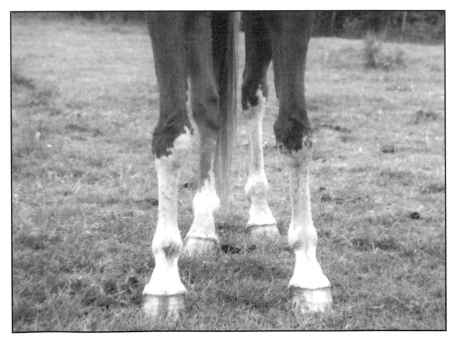

of ground beneath the foot. Thus a horse jumping down from a field onto a hard road is asking its limbs to absorb evident concussion to a degree that could easily end in injury. This concussion could almost be equalled by trotting fast along the same hard road.

Concussion is not only affected by condition of the surface, but also by fitness because exercise tends to strengthen and harden the body from the flaccid unfit state of the sedentary animal. An uneven, stony or pot-holed road may force the joints to take strain to one side or the other, bending them in a way that could cause injury. A steep camber may have the same effect. Excessively soft ground induces fatigue earlier and tends to cause tendon injuries, especially in animals whose fitness is in question.

The Hind Limb

For reasons already given, conformational and surface influences have a lesser effect on lameness in the hind limb, with the exception of the hock which is more commonly influenced by axial forces than any other joint in the limb.

Lameness is more common in the fore than hind limb. This is attrib-

Backward deviation of the knee is a common cause of lameness in horses. Forward deviation does not cause the same problems

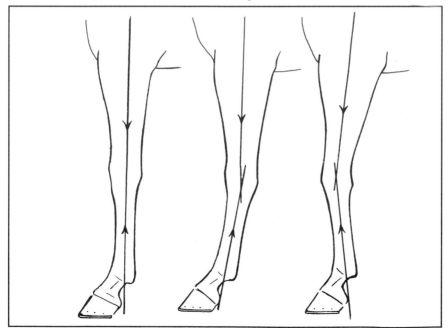

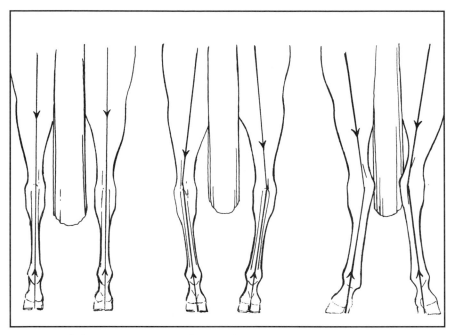

Anatomical deviations are equally significant in the hind limb; bone spavin is associated with poor conformation

uted to the weight-bearing function of the forelegs, particularly as these are subjected to a force estimated at many times the body weight when landing over a jump. Thus the bony and ligamentous structures of the foot, pastern, fetlock, cannon and knees are all exposed to direct concussive effects.

Hind limb lameness is more attributable to the spring-coil functions of the stifle and hock, and to the great muscle masses of the quarters and pelvis that help to raise the weight of the animal from the ground when required.

In practice, muscular injuries and disturbances of spinal column function are among the most common sources of lameness encountered today. This is very similar to the situation of the human athlete; the difference being that the human athlete is unable to perform with muscular or back pain whereas the horse is often expected to do so through ignorance of its suffering.

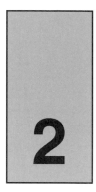

2 Diagnosis

Diagnosis of lameness will be discussed here in the context of facilities directly available to the ordinary horseowner and will only touch upon techniques which are within the strict domain of the specialist vet, e.g. radiography, diagnostic ultrasound, scintigraphy and other forms of bone and tissue scanning, and the procedure of nerve blocking.

It may be imagined that without these aids diagnosis is particularly cramped, but this is far from the case. The vast majority of lameness is diagnosed by the vet just as it is described here, by direct clinical examination, by intelligent observation, and by palpation and manipulation of the skeletal structures after the affected limb has been identified.

History

Taking the history of the problem is often of vital importance to lameness diagnosis, although it is sometimes fruitless and in many situations has to be disregarded. The following questions may be significant:

1) The owner's groom's opinion of the affected leg is important to the vet even though it may not be correct. Is there a possibility of more than one limb being involved?

2) What is the duration of the lameness and, if long standing, are the symptoms intermittent?

3) Is the lameness more noticeable on hard or soft ground; up or down hill?

4) Is it more noticeable when the horse is ridden? Some lamenesses will only be evident at this time.

5)   Is the lameness more prominent on one or other diagonal?
6)   Does the horse pull out lame?
7)   When the horse is warmed up does the lameness disappear?
8)   How is weight borne at rest? Is any limb favoured (i.e. held free of weight)?
9)   Any evident trauma, fall, kick, etc.?
10)   When was the horse last shod?

Locating the Limb Involved

The source of lameness is not always immediately apparent. The vet will take the following steps to locate the limb (or limbs) involved.
1)   The horse is first seen at rest in its stable and particular note taken of how weight is borne and if any limb is being favoured. When this is the case, and the affected limb is evident, examination of that limb can be started at once.
2)   If there is no evident abnormality, each of the hooves is picked out. While doing this, soreness, heat or some other symptoms of abnormality may be found in the foot itself. The horse's reluctance to raise a particular foot may indicate pain in another which will be forced to take added weight. Then the horse is taken outdoors. Standing square on level ground it is viewed from all sides looking for any tell-tale signs that might indicate which limb is affected. Of interest will be indications of pain in movement (especially when first coming out, any flinching when turning, or other suspect reactions as it is manoeuvred into place).
    Note is taken of evident swellings (particularly on joints or bones), and muscle wastage (especially in the neck, shoulders, back and quarters). Many swellings will take days to develop, depending on the underlying cause, and some established swellings are not necessarily associated with lameness. The degree of heat and pain will provide clues to their significance, although cold swellings may be the cause of lameness through impinging on other structures or altering action.
    An evident swelling may be the immediate cause of lameness, although an established splint (or an old sidebone, or ringbone, etc.) may not. Acute muscle injuries will usually result in local swelling and possible distortions of neighbouring anatomy due to fluid effusion, muscle spasm and pain.
    Attention is given to any evident swelling of joints, bursae, tendons, ligaments or sheaths. These are all soft swellings that occur in areas such as the fetlock, knee or hock; the tendons most often affected are the flex-

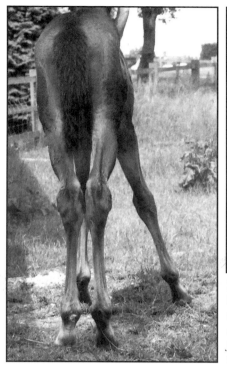
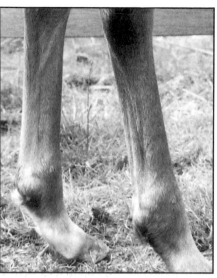

This foal (left and above) *is lame in the left hind limb and not bearing weight evenly on it. The fetlock and pastern are slightly dropped. The injury resulted from a fall and the foal recovered with rest*

This horse's knee (at left) *was enlarged as the result of a blow; there was no underlying bone damage*

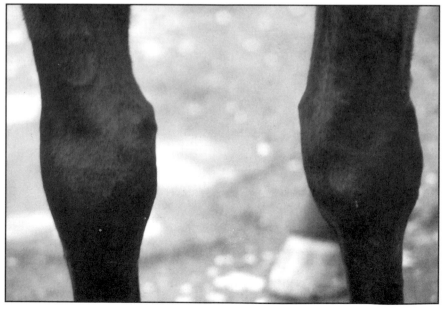

or tendons at the back of the cannon area in the forelimb. Bony swellings such as evident bucked shins or bone spavin are also noted.

The anatomy and structure of the vertebral column and related structures is particularly vital. Features of importance here are bony alignment, muscular spasm which might distort the shape of the spine, and areas of evident atrophy or swelling.

3)   After the full standing inspection, the horse is walked away and back in a straight line for a distance of 20-30m. Some abnormality may be

The horse is walked toward the examiner

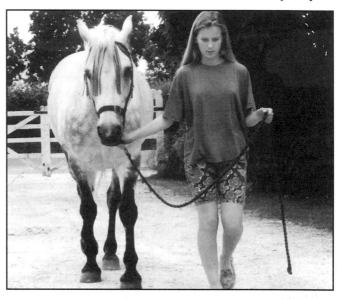

At the walk, watch for the level at hip, hock and foot

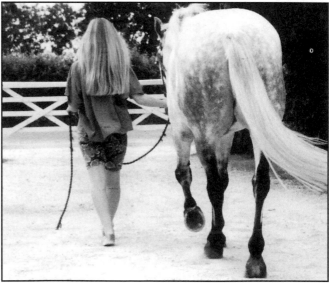

noticed now as the injured limb bears weight or as it moves through the air. These two distinct eventualities (weight-bearing and motion) immediately divide lameness into two basic types: supporting-leg lameness (pain indicated when the affected limb meets the ground) and swinging-leg lameness (pain when the affected limb is in motion). The importance of these two types of lameness is fundamental to diagnosis, because supporting-leg lameness normally indicates pain in the bony structures of the limb and/or their immediate soft tissue attachments. Swinging-leg lameness, on the other hand, is more commonly a sign of muscular or other soft tissue injury, or of pain emanating from the bony and soft tissue structures of the spine.

4)   When the horse comes back it is turned sharply to either side by the groom, ensuring that it is the horse that does the turning and not the groom. (This could alternatively be done after the horse has trotted.) This is achieved by the groom standing level with the centre of the horse on either side and making the animal turn its hind end away in a brisk and coordinated way for three or four full circuits. It is important that each limb moves freely without restriction and crosses over properly (i.e. the inner limb moving across the plane of the outer limb without difficulty). Where there is damage to, or interference with, spinal nerves, the horse may not be able to carry out this movement easily. Failure to do so could be an indication of conditions such as wobbling.

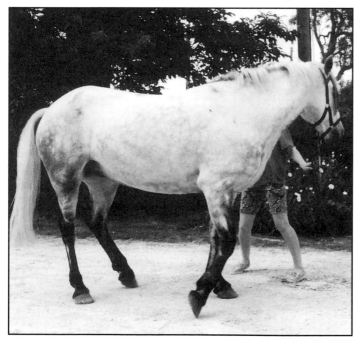

When the horse is turned sharply, the sequence of movements starts with the groom on the inside and the horse moving away from her

The turning sequence continues with the groom on the inside and the horse moving away from her, crossing the inner hind leg over the plane of the outer leg

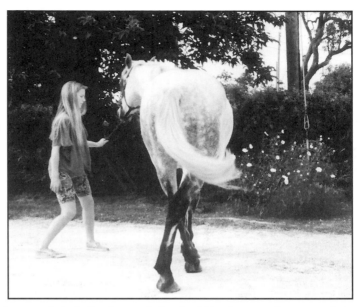

When turning is completed, the horse is backed for four or five complete strides, being asked to perform the exercise sharply and without objection. Again, where it fails to achieve this, suspicions might be aroused of pain in the back area or of nerve damage, but care must be taken to distinguish between inability and reluctance.

When the horse is backed its limbs must extend freely on either side

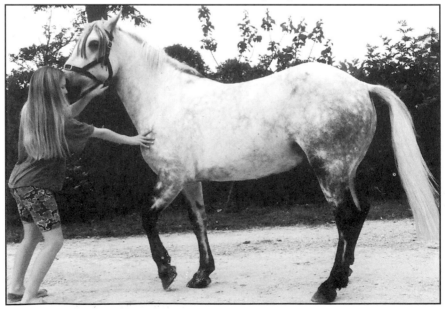

5)   The horse is now trotted away on a hard surface for much the same distance (20-30m) and its action carefully observed from behind. It is important to watch only the hind limbs at this point and to ignore the movement of the head because the head movement could be misleading where there is lameness to more than one limb.

Lameness, if present, will be marked at the trot; the groom must allow adequate rein for the horse's head to move freely, as in these two photographs

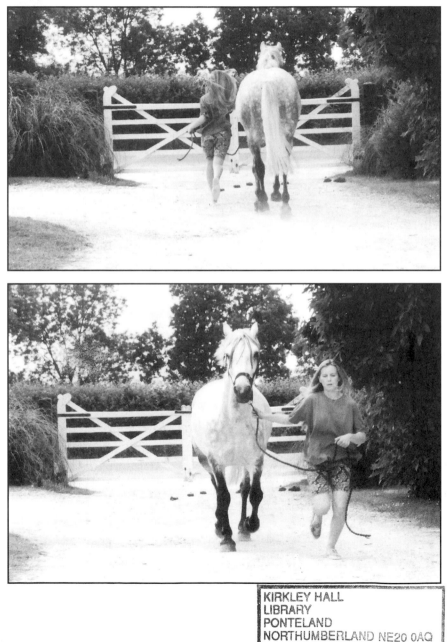

In supporting-leg lameness the hip of the affected hind limb will rise when the foot of that limb meets the ground. (Although we are deliberately ignoring the horse's head at this time to avoid confusion where there might be fore and hind limbs causing lameness, it actually drops at the same instant.) The opposite occurs with the sound limb.

While this single feature (movement at the level of the hip) is vital in detecting the affected limb, there are, it must be said, variations and degrees of abnormality, depending on the source of lameness and its severity. In some cases, the upper line of the quarter on the affected side may actually drop below normal as the limb is moved. This is common in swinging-leg lameness; pain being felt as the leg is in motion and so affecting the length and direction of stride in the process. While this may seem to confuse the issue it is easily distinguished with time and experience provided the front end of the horse is ignored as the animal moves away.

It is important to be able to eliminate the hind limbs as the probable source of lameness before the horse turns to come back. Where there is still doubt, the exercise can be repeated. The opinion of the animal's normal rider may also be of use at this time, as an added indication of whether impulsion has been lost from behind or if the lameness is in front. However, it must be appreciated that even the best riders can be confused,

The hips are level in a sound horse (left); *in supporting-leg lameness (right) the hip of the lame limb rises* (arrowed) *as the foot bears weight*

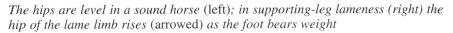
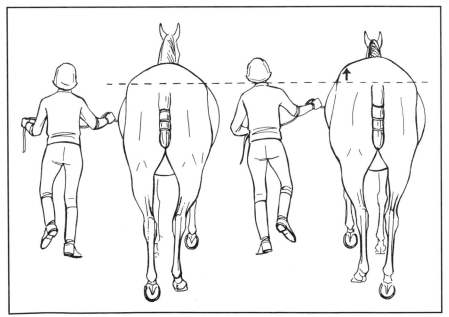

but their opinions are always valuable in cases of slight or intermittent lameness and can be of help in reaching a diagnosis.

It is also important, later, to view the action of the hind limbs from a side view, preferably viewing from each side separately. This can be done while observing the animal walk and trot on a straight line or on a lunge on a surface that is preferably not yielding. From this vantage point, the length of stride can be gauged as well as the action of the limb and the height to which each limb is raised from the ground while in motion.

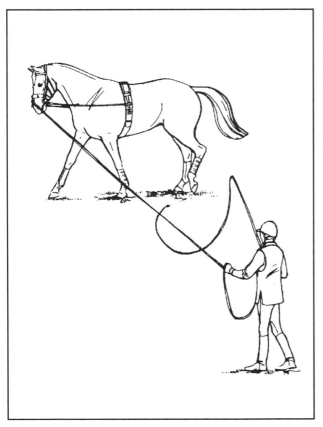

When lunged, the inner leg of the horse is likely to show increased lameness in supporting-leg lameness; the opposite may apply with muscular conditions because of tracking short

A horse is said to be not 'tracking up' properly when the length of stride varies (normally shorter on the affected side). However, the variation may be marginal and difficult to detect for any but the most experienced eye. Commonly, in muscular lameness the leg will appear to be fully extended but is retracted before actually striking the ground. The extension may appear normal to a point but there is a quick correction before the ground is struck. This in itself is abnormal but might not be easily detected if, for example, the horse is trotting in long grass.

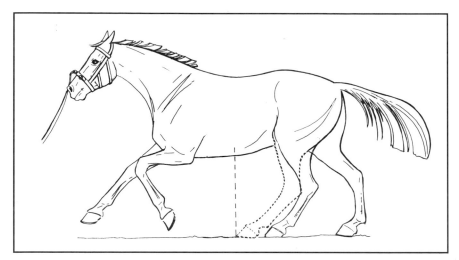

Failure to track-up behind occurs in lameness of joint, muscle or back origin: where the limb should extend to (dotted hind limb), as opposed to where it actually lands

It is also often easier to detect abnormal movement at hip and pelvic level when the horse is on the lunge and the affected limb is on the inner side of the circle. Again, it is wise to ignore the horse's head while examining the hind limb because its movements may only cause confusion.

Impaired flexion from the stifle and hock may be seen from this angle. But, as both joints move in unison, it is not easy to distinguish which is involved from observation at this distance.

Concussive lamenesses are more common in front than behind, and these are likely to be accentuated as the horse trots in a circle with the affected limb to the inside. It is important to be aware, however, that conditions resulting from loose or badly placed shoes may increase lameness at this time. These may produce direct pressure, say, on the site of corn, or, alternatively, a loose shoe may move inwardly and bring pressure to bear on the sensitive sole.

6)   When trotted straight back, a horse with supporting-leg lameness in the foreleg will show an upward movement of the head, occurring as the lame limb strikes the ground. The opposite applies to the sound limb.

With swinging-leg lameness this head movement again varies because the degree of upward movement may not be significant even though pain is felt as the affected limb is protracted forward. The pain is likely to alter the flight arc of the foot and may either cause a failure of the limb to be flexed to a normal height or there may be adduction or abduction as it moves through space.

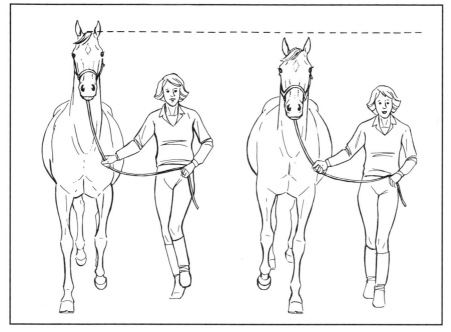

The head rises as the lame limb bears weight in supporting forelimb lameness. It does not in the normal horse

It should be appreciated that a bilateral peculiarity of movement may be conformational (therefore normal), but it could also be caused by bilateral lameness. Where it exists in only one limb, the chances are that there is lameness in that limb.

The movement of the head in weight-bearing lameness is intended to limit the amount of weight borne by the affected limb, and the time duration for which it is borne. Head movement when pain is felt during limb flight, on the other hand, is more likely to be due to compensation for stride deficiences, or as an effort to maintain balance.

7)   It is important to appreciate that lameness may exist in more than one limb at the same time and this will have a definite influence on movement at all gaits. Injuries may have resulted from distinct and separate incidents - they could also have occurred at the same time, or one might be secondary to the other. If both forelimbs are lame (as is possible with navicular disease), the stride is short and shuffling, but may be uniform on each side, and head movements are not pronounced.

In lameness originating from spinal structures, both front and hind limbs on a diagonal may be affected. This may be more pronounced under the weight of a rider.

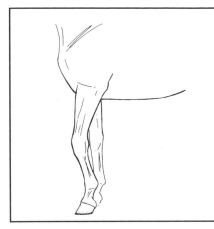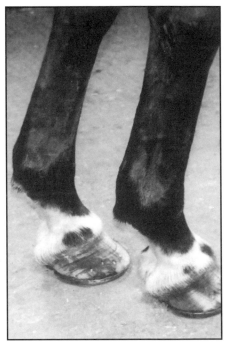

The animal's natural standing position (right) *which resulted from a fetlock injury. The right fore knee is forward and the fetlock more upright. Compare with the diagrammatic stance* (above)

When both hind limbs are affected (as in some cases of spavin), differences in movement of the two limbs may be difficult to detect.

8)   Secondary lameness is a very common feature in horses and often results from failure to detect primary minor lamenesses at an early stage. However, the initial lameness may cause an alteration in gait (quite often marginal in degree) which results in improper placement of the foot on that limb and this can expose other structures to injury, especially when the animal is travelling at speed or jumping. Many injuries to lower leg structures occur in this way and many continue to be aggravated until the primary source of the problem is located.

Secondary lameness occurs in the following situations:

a) As a result of dynamic changes in the upper limb causing improper placement of the foot.

b) As a result of improper weight distribution due to pain in a remote area (e.g. the pedal or navicular bone). Thus a fetlock may be strained because pain in the foot is being avoided.

c) Due to excessive weight being borne by a particular limb when compensating for pain in another (e.g. fracture, bad breakdown, etc.).

d) Muscle wastage occurs in some situations due to remote sources of pain (even when legs are in plaster casts) because the muscles of the limb are not being used.

However, this is not typical secondary lameness, even if the wasted muscle has to be encouraged back into use after the primary source has healed.

9)   In treating muscular injuries in horses which have had a hard season in competition, eventing, jumping or racing, it is not uncommon to detect injuries in limbs other than the one which is the source of an evident problem.

In some cases, two or even three limbs show evidence of muscular abnormality (as detected with Faradic-type muscle-stimulating equipment), as a consequence of one initial injury, through added strain on these remote structures. However, many of these animals are returned to full working normality with appropriate treatment.

Examination

Examination of the lame limb always begins at the foot. This is partly because the foot is a common source of lameness, but also because the examination has to be thorough and methodical.

The Foot

It is vital to inspect carefully the whole structure of the foot, both while it is resting on the ground and when picked up. First, it should be compared with its fellow, gauging the angles with the ground, with the line of the pastern and with the rest of the limb.

A healthy foot should not be contracted or boxy and the heel should be so constructed that the frog is fully expanded and in regular ground contact when the limb is in motion. At the coronet there should be no swelling of the type seen in low ringbone or buttress foot, and the wings of the cartilages should be soft and pliable at the level of the quarters (not solid as when ossified in sidebone). However, it must be appreciated that a foot can be abnormal visually (e.g. boxy, or contracted) and still not a source of lameness. The point is that evident abnormalities may or may not be the source; although, when examined for soundness, the same abnormalities may be considered likely to lead to lameness at a later stage.

The external hoof is felt by hand and examined for any evidence of pain or heat, which is best confirmed by comparison with its fellow. Heat is most common in foot infection, in fractures and in laminitis. Laminitis, however, is not usually confined to a single foot and heat will generally be found in other feet in this condition.

An odd-sized left foot. Compare with that on the opposite page

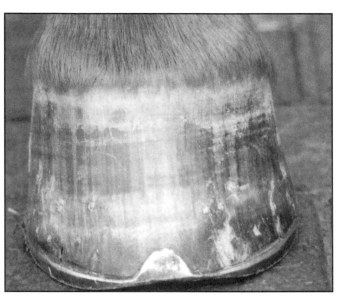

Next the foot is picked up and care taken to inspect the outline and lie of the shoe and to judge if it is tight or loose and whether or not the bearing surface is coming in contact with the sensitive sole. This is a critical factor in any lameness and it is also possible that a horse feeling pain from a shoe will alter its gait to avoid it and so endanger other areas.

A hoof tester may be used to bring pressure on various aspects of the foot in an effort to determine and localise pain. This is best done in a methodical manner, first checking the full circumference of the wall and the area of each nail in particular. Next the bars, frog and the surface over the navicular bone (junction of middle and posterior thirds of the foot) are subjected to directly applied pressure in sequence.

It is particularly important to check the heels at the level of the coronet (even using finger pressure only) because pus often accumulates there. This may be marked by swelling, by pale discoloration of the coronet itself, and may make the area sensitive to any kind of handling.

Pain, as a response to any of these procedures, is usually marked by an effort to pull the limb away. However, it is important to be wholly objective in assessing this because some animals may pull away for secondary reasons and this would have to be appreciated. Vets always repeat the exercise and ensure that any reaction is a direct result of the application of pressure. They may also tap firmly (but not excessively) over the ends of the individual nails to check for pain. While the hoof is on the ground the wall may be tapped for the same reason. If there is any doubt, the reaction can be compared with that found in a sound foot.

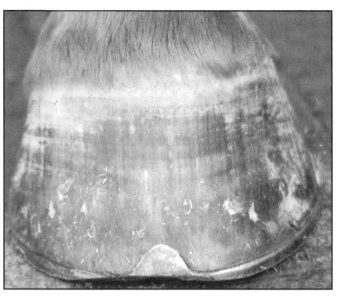

The right foot of the same horse, working sound

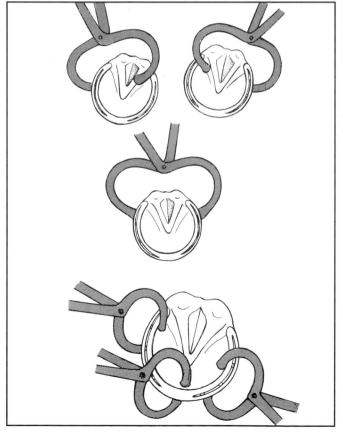

Using a hoof tester: the full circumference of the wall is examined first (below); *then each side of the frog* (top); *and finishing with examination* (centre) *of the navicular area*

These feet have lost their shape as a result of laminitis. Note the broken foot/pastern axis

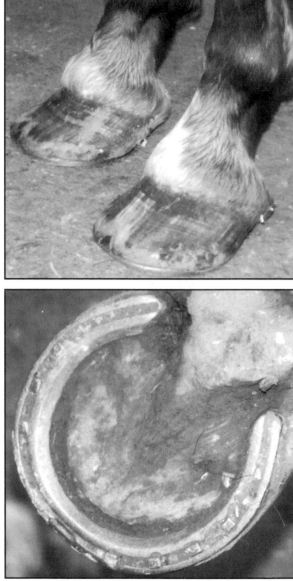

The sole of this foot has dropped and the farrier has dug a trench to avoid sole pressure with the shoe

If it appears that foot lameness is present, it is usual to have the shoe removed so that the examination can be taken further.

The Rest of the Limb

If the foot has been eliminated as a source of lameness the rest of the affected limb is examined methodically from the ground upwards. The

signs sought are heat, swelling, atrophy, constriction, or pain in any structure examined.

Heat

There is a sensitive form of thermometer now available for heat detection
(thermography) and although the instrument may be advantageous in the
right hands, it can lead to misinterpretation, so heat is best detected manually with the palm of the hand. It is a facility that is perfected with practice, through constant observation (to detect abnormal areas) and regular
handling of limbs. Racehorse trainers tend to be adept at it, and gain their
experience by handling numerous tendons and fetlocks in particular

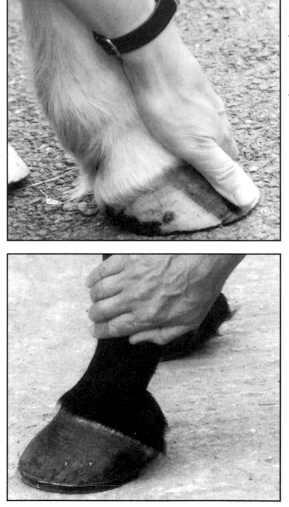

*Feeling for heat is carried
out using the palm and the
fingers. The vet is feeling
various areas of the horse's
limbs: here* (left) *the coronet and hoof;* (below) *the
fetlock and sesamoids*

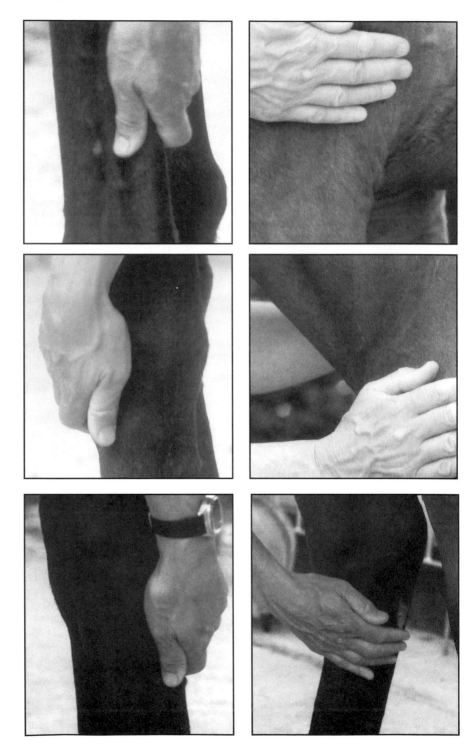

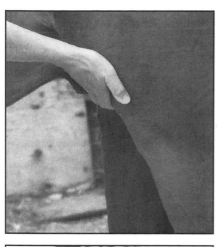

Feeling for heat (from top left, clock-wise)*: the upper tendon area; over the elbow joint; over the shoulder joint; over the seat of spavin; at the back of the knee; on the front of the knee*

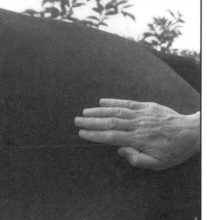

THIS PAGE
Feeling for heat (above)*: over the stifle joint; and* (left) *over the hip joint*

throughout their years with horses. The same knowledge is available to any person who is in daily contact with a number of horses.

Swelling
Swellings on limbs are found easily with a good knowledge of surface anatomy. These swellings may be soft, as in bursal, sheath and joint inflammation; or hard, as with bony exostoses, as occur in ringbone or bucked shins. (With sore shins there may be no evident swelling, but the front of the cannon is extremely sensitive to touch.)

Atrophy
Atrophy (or wasting) is most easily seen in larger muscle groups, and is particularly common in the shoulder region. It is marked by shrinking of

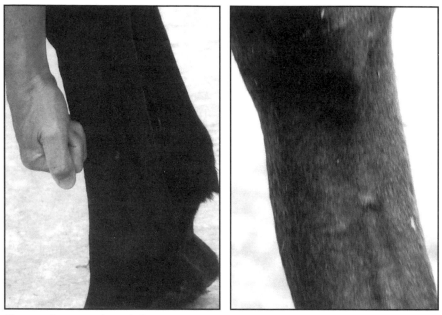

Testing for sore shins (left)*; a quick, firm movement will cause an affected horse to flinch. The swelling* (right) *at the front of the leg is called a 'bucked shin'*

Muscle atrophy in the scapular region

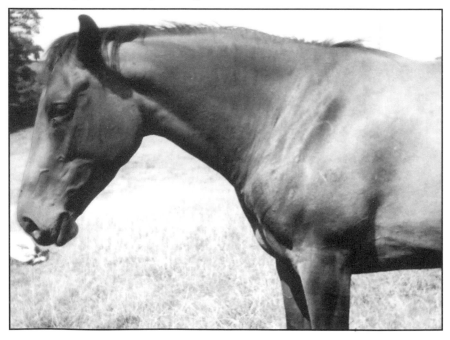

the muscle body and is recognised by the loss of normal conformation. This may best be established by comparison with the same muscle area of the other limb (it would be unusual to find the same muscle atrophied on both limbs).

Constriction

Constriction occurs on occasion in the annular ligament of the fetlock, most commonly at the back of the joint where the superficial tendon passes through a ring formed by the deep tendon; or at the back of the knee (in carpal tunnel injury).

Pain

The presence of pain in individual structures is generally detected through manipulation or movement of that structure and interpretation of the animal's reaction. This does not have to involve violent force, which may only have the effect of making matters worse. As with a hoof tester, the amount of pressure applied to the part only has to be adequate, very slight in many cases. There is no justification for being rough or crude in this examination.

The Forelimb

In examining individual areas of the forelimb the vet will follow the procedure, already mentioned, of working from the ground upwards.

The Pastern

Swellings or inflammation of the pastern are most notably seen in low (at the coronet) or high (mid-pastern) ringbone. Heat may be detected around either of these two regions (without swelling) which roughly represents the coffin and pastern joints respectively. Injury in either location would normally be accompanied by marked lameness and if the condition were chronic there would usually be bony enlargement. However, it is possible for established ringbone lesions to settle down and for affected horses to be functionally sound.

Any of the soft tissue structures at the back of the pastern may be injured: the superficial and deep flexor tendons, the sesamoidean ligaments and the digital synovial sheath. These injuries must not be confused with swelling caused by ascending infection of the foot or the type of filling that accompanies conditions such as lymphangitis. Swelling at the front of the pastern may also be caused by injury to the common digital extensor tendon and its attachments to the pedal bone.

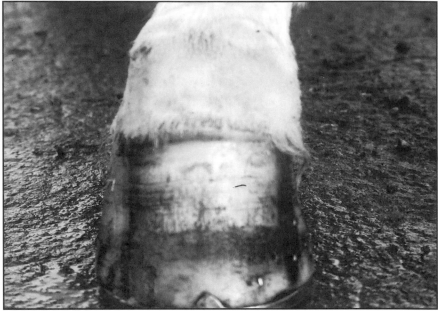

The low ringbone growth here is most prominent on the outer part of the limb

Extensive low ringbone formation with pressure on the coronet, causing hoof growth defects

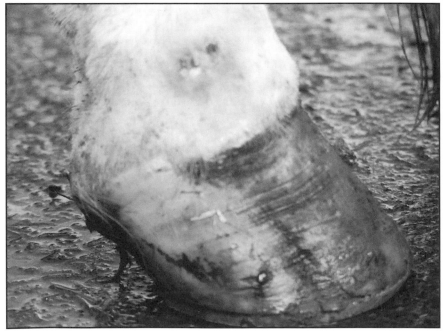

Heat in any part of the pastern area may also be accompanied by pain on gentle movement of associated structures. It could be localised as in strain of the pastern joint or its ligaments.

If it is certain that the source of lameness is identified here, and there is no localised infection involved, the area may have to be radiographed later. However, it is still important to eliminate any other source of lameness in the limb.

The Fetlock

When assessing the fetlock we include the proximal sesamoid bones.

Swelling of the fetlock may be hard or soft in nature, involving either bone or soft tissue structures. Soft swellings are common at the back of the joint and may involve the digital sheath or the palmar (posterior) extension of the fetlock joint capsule. These are both called windgalls, which are generally of little significance as a cause of lameness; however, their significance would be treated with greater concern if there were pain and heat in the region, as with a recent strain to these or other local structures.

Heat is particularly significant at the back of the joint over the proximal sesamoid bones. Fractures of these bones, or disruptions of their ligamentous attachments, are a common cause of chronic lameness. While heat may be relatively simple to detect over the sesamoids, there may be little or no swelling, but lameness is usually marked, especially when the horse is turning. Horses with chronic sesamoiditis, however, especially if confined for some days before examination, may pull out almost sound and the heat in the region may be so slight it could be missed easily.

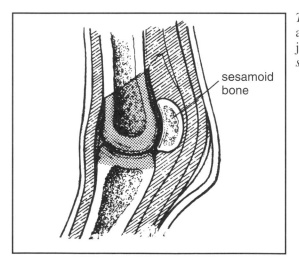

sesamoid bone

The fetlock joint (the tinted area shows the extent of the joint capsule) *with sesamoid bone adjacent*

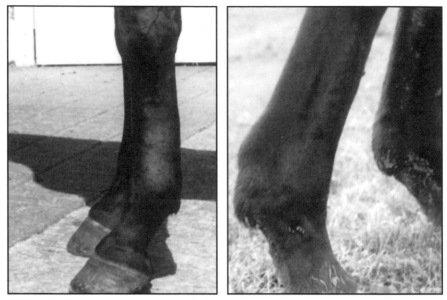

Filling (left) *can be seen over the fetlock, with a slight bow at the back of the tendons in the mid-cannon area.* *Chronic swelling* (right) *over the tendons just above the fetlock*

Swelling of the joint itself may follow acute strain and is marked by pain, heat and severe lameness.

The bony element of the fetlock may enlarge over a period due to excessive concussion and is often an indication of degenerative joint disease (DJD, also called osteoarthritis). This condition is most commonly found in young horses trained for two-year-old racing and is an extremely serious problem with regard to the animal's future prospects.

DJD should not be confused with enlargement of the lower growth plate of the third metacarpal (cannon) that occurs in foals. This latter condition (normally called epiphysitis, or, more recently, physitis) is not necessarily of great concern. It can occur when foals are growing strongly, when the ground is hard in mid-summer, or when there is disturbance of nutritional balance (mostly involving calcium, phosphorus and vitamin D). In some cases the condition can become clinical, but most foals grow through it without serious complication as long as diet and exercise are duly controlled.

The Cannon Area
Lameness related to the cannon area is most commonly caused by injuries to the tendons or ligaments at the back of the leg or to the bony structures (the second, third and fourth metacarpal bones) themselves.

Tendon injuries are most common in the superficial flexor, but can also occur in the deep flexor tendon beneath it, or in the inferior check ligament which attaches the deep flexor to the annular ligament of the carpal joint.

The suspensory ligament, a vital part of the stay apparatus that allows the horse to rest while standing, is commonly injured at the level of the sesamoid bones or a short distance above them. All these injuries display heat and pain in the early stages and swelling usually develops quickly, depending on the severity of the injury.

The front of the cannon bone is the site of sore shins. As already stated, this may or may not be associated with marked swelling of the bone itself, but it is a very painful condition that is most common in young horses.

Splints occur between the small and large metacarpal bones in the ligament that attaches each splint bone to the cannon and in the small

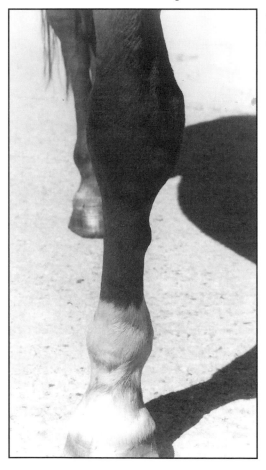

Splints are most common on the inside of the forelimb
(Photo: Sue Devereux)

metacarpal (splint) bones themselves. They are usually marked by prominent bony swellings which are easily detected on the inner (more often) or outer side of the limb. They generally do not cause lameness when fully developed. Conversely, very small splints which are sensitive to the touch are often a source of lameness.

The Knee

Heat or swelling in the knee (carpus) is associated with a number of conditions caused by injury to the small bones themselves and the ligaments that bind them together. Swelling without heat may result from superficial injuries to the surface of the knee or from chronic injuries to the bony structures.

The conformation of the knee may provide clues to the source of the injury. For example, if the horse is naturally back at the knee injury to bones is a real prospect.

Synovial swellings may occur in the sheaths of tendons which cross the knee, such as the long digital extensor at the front or the carpal sheath and sheath of the *flexor carpi radialis* at the back. Most of these swellings can occur in the absence of lameness, so their presence has to be evaluated objectively.

Swellings of the ligaments binding the knee may exist as a chronic

Bony enlargement on the front of a pony's knee

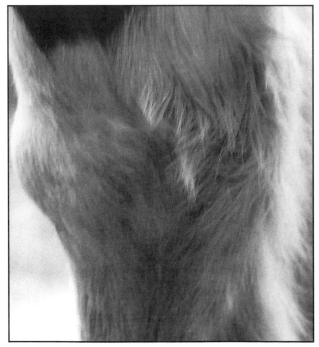

reminder of an earlier serious knee injury. However, their influence in joint movement has to be assessed, because it is possible for horses to perform and jump soundly even in the presence of such swellings.

The knee, being such a complex structure, very often has to be radiographed to identify the exact source of lameness. However, it is generally possible to pinpoint it as the likely source by external signs only.

The Forearm and Elbow
Gross features of abnormality on the forearm are not that common, although fractures of the radius or ulna do occur. With any physical injury to this part there may be swelling, or atrophy, of muscle; and the lower epiphysis of the radius is often enlarged in young horses creating the condition called 'open knees'.

The point of the elbow may be enlarged (capped elbow) and this is marked by a bursal enlargement that may contain varying amounts of fluid, or infection. Separation of the attachments between the radius and

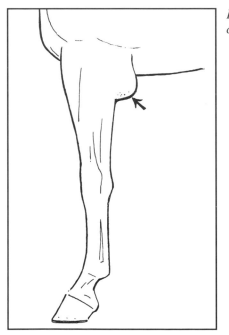

Position of swelling (arrowed) *in capped elbow*

ulna is also known and this is responsible for a supporting-leg lameness that is persistent but not always very marked.

The Shoulder Area
Injury of the shoulder joint itself is not very usual in mature horses, but

injury to muscles in this area is a regular feature of modern equine lameness. Many such injuries are not diagnosed until chronic and this very often leads to the involvement of other structures which have compensated for the pain in the affected muscle. On manual examination, muscle injury is detected by intimate knowledge of the anatomy of the region and is marked by atrophy, or swelling, and by the detection of changes within the substance of the muscle itself. Muscle, which is nomally elastic and pliable, in these cases can be hard and gritty with evident areas of abnormality found.

Bursitis at the front of the shoulder joint (marked by soft swelling) is commonly recorded and bony injuries may occur in the same region as a result of striking doors, etc.

The pectoral muscles at the front and inner side of the limb at this point are also frequently damaged and evident changes can best be detected by comparison with the other side.

The Withers

At the withers, a common cause of swelling in the past was inflammation of the bursa that lies between the vertebral spines and the *ligamentum nuchae* (fistulous withers). (In the United Kingdom and Ireland, this condition has reduced in incidence since the virtual elimination of brucellosis from the national cattle herds.)

Pain in the withers area is also common from galls caused by poorly-fitting saddles, but it may also indicate spinal origin lameness due to minor disturbances in the vertebral column.

Fracture of the dorsal spinous processes might be indicated by acute pain on handling. This injury could happen through a fall.

The Neck and Back

Neck pain is commonly a result of muscle injuries sustained in training or of pressure on spinal nerves as they emerge from between the vertebrae (one of these could ensue from the other). Its presence is seen as restriction of natural movement and inhibited flexion to either side, or up and down.

The dorsal surface of the horse's back is subject to injuries resulting from locomotion that causes primary muscle damage, or disturbance to the vertebrae themselves. This may be reflected in altered gait at the walk and trot and may also cause anatomical changes which are relatively simple to identify. The dorsal line of the vertebral spine should be level and straight (but it is important not to confuse abnormality with roach, or

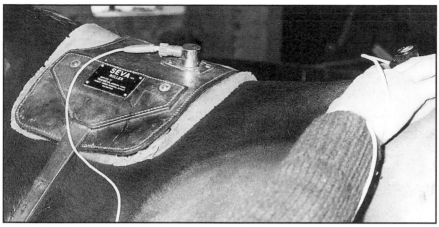

Treatment of muscular injury of the horse's back involves Faradism. Here the indifferent electrode is strapped to the back and the active electrode stimulates reaction in the treatment area   (Photo: Stuart Newsham)

dipped, back, both of which are perfectly natural anatomy, if less than ideal).

Muscular spasm, resulting from minor mechanical disruptions of bony alignment, may alter the shape of the back and tend to pull the spine marginally to one side or the other. Disruption of the sacroiliac joint between the sacrum and ilium is not uncommon, particularly in jumping horses.

This pony has a dipped back as a result of old age

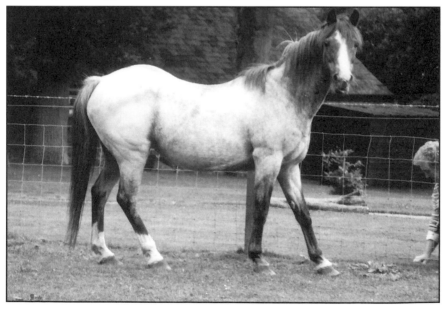

This may be marked in chronic cases by muscle wastage in the gluteal region above the pelvis and by unevenness of the pelvic profile when viewed from behind.

The Hind Limb

From the ground to the hock the anatomy of the hind limb is similar in most details to the forelimb and while conditions causing lameness are not as common, they do occur. Thus injuries to the flexor tendons are not seen to the same extent, and conditions like navicular disease are seldom recorded.

The Hock

Soft swellings on the hock are referred to as bog spavin when the joint capsule itself is enlarged. The distension of the joint is most evident at the anteromedial (inside front) aspect, and also behind, on either side, at the level of the depression in front of the point of the hock.

Bone spavin occurs on the inner side of the hock and is located

Bone spavin occurs on the inner and lower side of the hock
(Photo: Sue Devereux)

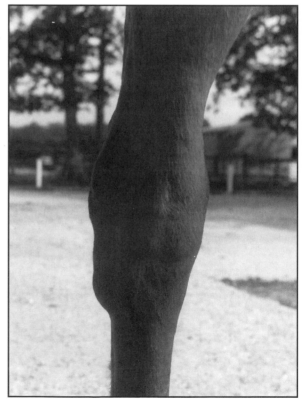

between the proximal and distal rows of tarsal bones and between the lower row of tarsal bones and the large metatarsal (cannon) bone. The swelling here results from DJD and may be extensive. If there are no obvious signs or swelling, the condition is called occult spavin.

Thoroughpin is a soft tissue swelling behind and above the hock on either side and involves the tarsal sheath which encloses the deep flexor tendon.

Curb occurs at the lower extremity of the hind surface of the hock, immediately above the back of the cannon bone.

The Gaskin

The same applies to the gaskin as to the forearm of the front limb: injury here is not common except as a consequence of direct external impacts. The tibia may suffer fracture from kicks and this would normally be associated with considerable damage to muscles in the region.

The Stifle

The stifle is commonly a source of lameness and is very often associated with synovial distension of the joint. Injury may involve any of the anatomical structures that make up the joint.

Lameness may also ensue quite dramatically with upward fixation of the patella, when the patella locks on the medial trochlea of the femur.

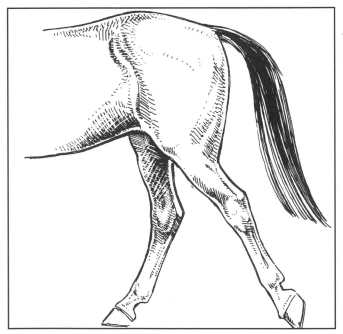

In upward fixation of the patella, the limb is locked in extension

This may occur at rest or at the walk and is often associated with upright conformation of the stifle joint.

Stifle lameness may also be a result of rupture to the cruciate ligaments of the joint, allowing abnormal movement of the joint, backwards and forwards, in a standing position.

The Hip

The hip joint is deeply situated and not a common source of lameness, being protected to a great extent by the strength of its anatomical construction. Heat over the joint is difficult to detect on surface examination.

Muscular injury in the region of the hip and stifle is common as is injury at the back of this area in the muscles extending down from the pelvis.

Surface and Gradient in Lameness

It is surprising how many marginally lame horses show increased signs on uneven surfaces, not from stones contacting the sole but simply from trotting up or down hill. All these factors have their own importance in the diagnosis of lameness. Horses with splints and sore shins are often more lame trotting down hill on a firm surface, while those with muscular problems may be far worse when climbing a soft bank. Similarly, muscular

Trotting down hill increases lameness in sore shins and splints

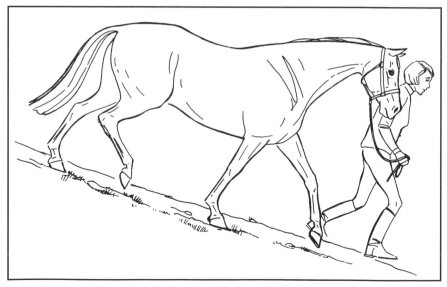

injuries can have serious implications for swimming horses. Failure to appreciate this can lead to accidents, because horses with back injuries are often unable to swim and there is, therefore, a risk of drowning.

Flexion Tests

It is a fundamental fact of lameness that movement of injured structures causes pain. This is conveyed by the horse through efforts to avoid pain by pulling the limb away, and the strength of this effort is often directly proportional to the extent of the pain felt.

Pain, it must be understood, is a protective mechanism which ensures rest for injured structures and so allows time for repair. It is a beneficial reaction, not simply an inconvenience, and its suppression (through the use of drugs or other means) can leave weakened areas open to more serious injury. This should never be forgotten.

The purpose of flexion tests is to expose covert lameness by subjecting structures of individual joints to prolonged flexing (anything from one

The degree of flexion will vary, but no flexion test should ever, of itself, make a horse go lame

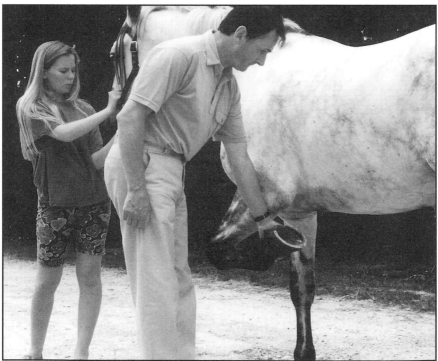

half to two minutes). This, it is hoped, will expose lameness not already evident and accentuate lameness of minor intensity. It is also used as a means of identifying the specific joint that is causing trouble.

The limitations of the exercise reside in the difficulty of flexing almost any joint without having an indirect effect on others. For example, flexion of the hock automatically involves flexion of the stifle - because of the reciprocal apparatus - and flexing any limb for two minutes places an added stress not only on the weight-bearing limb, but also on other structures such as the back and associated muscles.

A further criticism of flexion is that when carried out for too long a period it too can be a source of lameness.

However, having laid out these limitations, the exercise is still used as a standard part of lameness diagnosis and is found helpful in experienced hands.

Nerve Blocks

The use of nerve blocks enables clinicians to relate the source of lameness to specific anatomical structures. It is a specialised technique, requiring detailed knowledge of anatomy, and should not be practised by unskilled hands.

Nor should it be used routinely until the whole limb has been examined and the general area causing the problem has been identified.

To use nerve blocks as a means of eliminating specific areas with no detectable change is a suspect clinical tactic that is not always justified.

Examination of the Muscular System

Examination of muscles is carried out routinely when no evident source of lameness is found on the horse's lower limb structures, or when evident deformity in specific muscles is detected visually. Even where a gross lesion of, say, the fetlock or tendon, exists it is always important to know whether or not these have arisen as a result of some less obvious remote injury.

Chronic tendon lesions are frequently associated with long-standing shoulder muscle injury. These will not respond to normal therapies unless the muscle injury is first corrected. The same applies to many other lower limb injuries.

Muscular examination is carried out first visually, then manually.

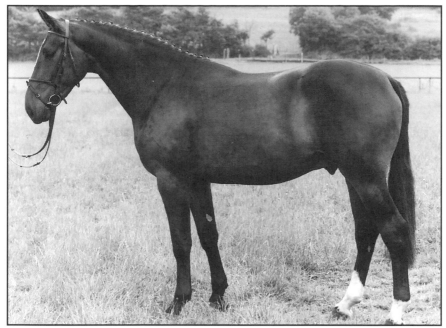

The profile of the horse's back is ideally free-flowing without any deviations, breaks in natural contour or evident muscle abnormality (Photo John Birt)

Finally, a Faradic-type muscle stimulator may be used; such equipment is extremely effective in testing muscle normality and identifying injured areas.

Back Manipulation

Manipulation of the back, part of the field of chiropractic, is a developing feature of animal therapy which receives a certain amount of scepticism from within professional circles. However, it is increasingly appreciated by all those intimately involved with performance horses, that pain and lameness associated with spinal structures is extremely common and that manipulation affords an effective means of correction in a high percentage of cases.

The source of the problem is identified by manual examination of the external surface of the vertebral column. Correction of identified abnormalities is done by swift precise movements that alter alignment and relieve muscle spasm as well as possibly easing unwanted pressure on emerging spinal nerves.

Location of the Injured Area

Having identified the limb, certain features of movement will assist location of the injured area.

The Shoulder

When in motion, the affected limb is not extended as far forward as the sound limb. The toe may be dragged and the neck muscles are more obviously used to assist forward movement of the limb. At rest, the limb may be flexed with the toe resting on the ground.

The Elbow

In movement, when the elbow is involved, weight is taken first by the toe with the knee slightly flexed. At rest, the elbow may be dropped and the knee and fetlock flexed when the limb is not bearing weight.

The Knee

In severe lameness relating to the knee joint, the limb is held flexed at rest, with the knee itself bearing little weight. Lameness is usually acute at the trot.

However, even with some minor fractures, weight may be borne when resting, and lameness is not marked at first if the animal has been rested for a few days.

The Cannon

The most common forms of lameness in the cannon are caused by splints or sore shins.

Splints
The affected limb may be carried further out from the body than its fellow while trotting, this being done to lessen the weight borne by the painful area.

Sore Shins
A short choppy step may be accompanied by the horse standing over at the knee. Some animals with sore shins anticipate the pain of handling and will lift the limb from the ground when approached.

The Pastern

The most common cause of lameness in the pastern area, aside from fractures, is caused by ringbone formation; the stride is shortened and the lameness is accentuated on turning. However, when the condition has settled, the animal may be functionally sound, but with an altered gait.

The Foot

Several sources of lameness are common in the foot.

Corn

The horse will try to relieve pressure on the affected part by raising the heel and shortening the forward phase of the stride. This same principle applies to any other source of foot pain.

Navicular Disease

There is a short stride with marked lameness, which, in the earlier stages of the disease, may disappear with exercise.

The Hip

There is shortening of the stride with the toe striking the ground first. The haunch on the affected side is lifted notably. This might best be seen with the horse trotting on a circle.

The Stifle

The stride is shortened and the toe inclines laterally. At rest the joint is flexed. Swelling may be evident at the front of the joint.

The Hock

Improper extension of the affected leg and dragging of the toe when moving is suggestive of conditions such as spavin. However, similar signs may arise from improper function of the axial spine.

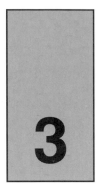

3 Concussive Lameness

This chapter deals with any lameness in which axial forces are a common precipitating factor.

While it is possible that some conditions placed in other categories could also be classified here, the point of the exercise is to stress the importance of this cause of lameness so that constructive efforts are made in future to limit its effect.

As no specific concussive conditions occur above the knee (although the structures above the knee can be influenced by consussive lameness) this joint will be used as a starting point, working down the limb.

Carpal Injuries (Carpitis)

The carpus, or knee, of the horse is a complex structure consisting of three distinct articulations:

1)   The radiocarpal joint formed between the lower end of the radius and the upper row of carpal bones (capable of opening to the extent of 90 degrees).

2)   The intercarpal joint formed between the two rows of carpal bones (capable of opening to 70 degrees).

3)   The carpometacarpal joint formed between the lower row of carpal bones and the upper ends of the metacarpal bones (does not open).

The equine knee corresponds to the human wrist. There are usually seven carpal bones, but sometimes eight, arranged in two rows one above the other. The bones of the upper row are: radial carpal, intermediate

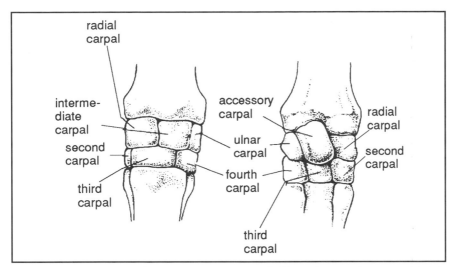

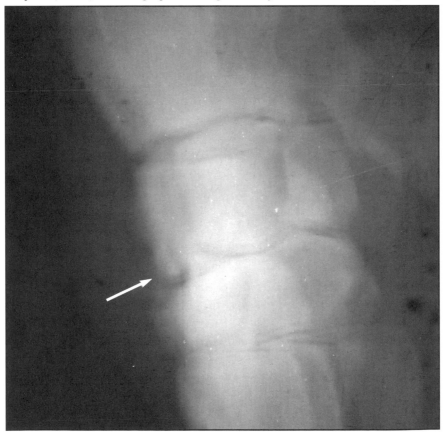

Bones of the carpus (above): *anterior view* (left) *and posterior view* (right).
Carpitis (below): *a radiograph showing a small fracture and new bone growth*

carpal, ulnar carpal, and the accesssory carpal at the back. Those of the lower row are: first carpal, second carpal, third carpal and fourth carpal.

Definition
Injuries to the knee involve disruption of the joint (or joints); tearing of the ligaments, or damage to the bones that constitute it.

Causes
The knee is an essential structure in the absorption of axial forces caused by ground contact and body weight. Conformation dictates absorption ability although even good natural conformation can be subjected to abnormal stresses due to fatigue at the end of an extended gallop or race. Some of the weight-bearing load is taken by the intercarpal ligaments and by displacement of the carpal bones to either side. The capacity to transfer the burden in this way is developed with training, so that if training proceeds too fast the risk of injury increases.

The knee absorbs these forces and ideally transfers their passage upwards or down through the limb. At the point of weight bearing, the cannon, knee and radius are locked in the form of a rigid strut, which means that no individual structure bears an undue burden under normal circumstances. However, this changes with poor conformation as well as fatigue. Abnormal forces may be applied to individual bones or ligaments in these latter situations causing immediate inflammation, or, ultimately, degenerative joint disease (DJD).

At the end of a race, the knee may deviate backwards, increasing the risk of injury to the carpal bones

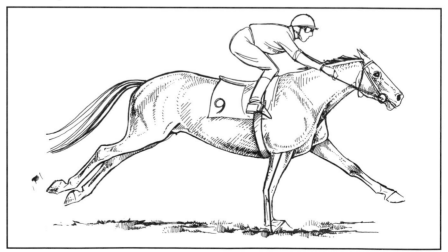

The knee may also be influenced by foot balance. Thus a long toe, low heel combination may alter the angulation of the cannon/knee/radius complex and thus encourage injury. A high heel and a short toe reduces the capacity of the foot to absorb axial forces and so places a greater load on all other weight-bearing structures.

Signs
There is swelling of the front of the knee with heat and pain on palpation. Lameness is generally marked, but chronically affected animals may show only slight signs and may knuckle on trotting, especially on uneven surfaces. The swelling is soft and tense with recent injuries, because of a marked increase of synovial fluid and there is usually heat on palpation. Bony enlargement may be evident in more chronic cases.

Radiographs are essential in any chronic swelling of the knee to eliminate the possibility of bone fractures and chips.

Treatment
Lasers and ultrasound are commonly used to relieve the symptoms and reduce inflammation of the joint. These forms of therapy are remarkably effective in conditions of recent origin, and may even help to promote repair of small bone fragments if the leg is kept immobilised.

However, it is important that treatment be commenced when the injury is fresh and before chronic changes in the joint structures have developed. Drugs such as sodium hyaluronate and polysulphated glycosaminoglycan (PSGAG) influence the restoration of normal joint function and often prove significant in the absence of fractures and advanced joint disease.

The modern surgical approach to carpal joint injuries involves arthroscopy, where the interference to the joint is minimal and removal of chips and other diseased tissues is possible through very small incisions. The arthroscope allows visual examination of the joint, and the procedure is often accompanied by irrigation to flush out damaged tissues and remove infectious material.

Splints

The small metacarpal (and metatarsal) bones are commonly known as splint bones.

Definition
Splints are bony enlargements that develop between a small and large

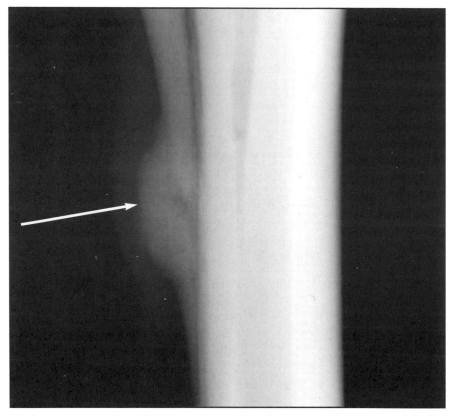

Radiograph showing splint formation with underlying small metacarpal (splint bone) fracture

metacarpal (or metatarsal) bone and frequently involve the smaller bone itself. They are most commonly seen on the inner side of the forelimb but may occur at the junction between these bones in any limb. The splint bones are attached to the large metacarpal/metatarsal by ligament. This ligament ossifies in later years but this does not prevent the development of splints in older animals.

A splint is created by the disturbance of the ligament and new bone growth. On radiograph, it is not unusual to find fractures of the splint bone involved in splint formation.

Definition
There are some distinct situations in which splints develop.
1)   In the young developing animal, especially at the yearling stage, when being fed heavily for sales.

2)   When store horses are being broken and ridden. In this situation, conformation is very often a factor.
3)   In older competing horses when foot balance has changed through ageing or bad shoeing.
4)   In animals of any age with poor limb conformation.

Splints are associated with poor foot/limb balance in a high percentage of cases, and it is probable that they occur as a result of the effect of this on axial forces. Their influence and size are often reduced by corrective shoeing and proper foot trimming.

Any change of limb axis that brings pressure to bear on a single splint bone is likely to result in splints. This could, quite simply, be trauma, but is also a common result of bad shoeing in which foot balance is lost through improper trimming. Downward pressure from the knee on to the splint bones can also cause splints, and may have the same basic cause of incorrect foot balance.

Splint development may indicate a combination of factors (nutritional as well as conformational), particularly in younger horses. Problems affecting the formation of bone also play a part, (i.e. deficiencies of vitamin A, D and E, calcium, magnesium, and phosphorus).

Signs
Splints are seen as hard bony swellings found between the splint and cannon bones; they may be single or numerous, small or extensive. Their position in relation to the knee and suspensory ligament is important because interference with the movement of either of these structures may prove a serious complication of the condition.

Initially, splint lameness is associated with heat and pain on palpation in the region of the developing growth. There may be little or no swelling at this stage although supporting-leg lameness is seen at the trot.

Large, developed splints may be hard and cold to the touch, free of pain on palpation, and the animal may not be lame. Some animals, usually owing to conformation, have a propensity to multiple splint development. There may be intermittent low-grade lameness, but the condition can be helped by corrective shoeing.

Lameness from splints is aggravated on rough ground or when a horse is asked to trot down hill. The affected limb may be splayed outwards from the body in movement.

By lifting the leg, with the knee flexed, a splint may be felt outside the suspensory ligament, in the region of the splint bone. It should be noted that many animals show varying degrees of sensitivity to being handled and a distinction needs to be made between this and true pain when deciding on the significance of any lesion.

Some large splints that develop suddenly in young horses do not cause lameness, but others that are barely visible frequently do.

Radiographs may help with diagnosis and will also help to eliminate the possibility of a fracture.

Treatment
In younger horses, rest will encourage the splint to harden. It is vital to ensure that the balance of the feet is attended to and that the diet is normal.

Using anti-inflammatory drugs in this condition is generally unnecessary. The cause has to be established and rectified; if it is a nutritional problem, the animal may become sound when the diet is corrected, but the splint may remain for life. Where the splint is due to faulty foot care, correction may well see it regress quickly.

Blistering and firing of splints has commonly been done, but there is no evidence to indicate that either advances the healing process in any way. The condition responds to corrective shoeing better than to any other form of therapy.

Sore and Bucked Shins

The shin is the area between the carpus and fetlock at the front of the limb, representing the front of the large metacarpal (or cannon) bone.

Definition
This is an inflammation of the periosteum (the outer covering) of the large metacarpal and metatarsal bones often associated with microfracture of the bone itself. It is more common in the fore than hind legs. When, in extreme cases, there is swelling of the front of the bone, the condition is described as 'bucked shin'

Causes
The problem is most common in two- and three-year-old horses trained for Flat racing and is probably an expression of immaturity combined with concussion. It also occurs in young National Hunt horses before maturity, which may not be fully achieved until six years of age.

It usually occurs as a result of working on hard ground but also appears regularly when the surface is sticky or holding and this may be due to

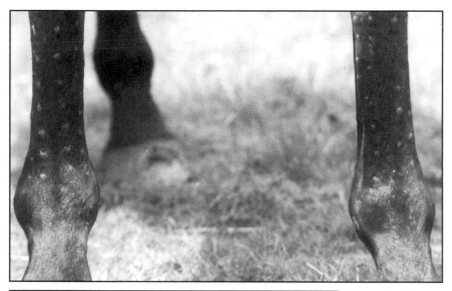

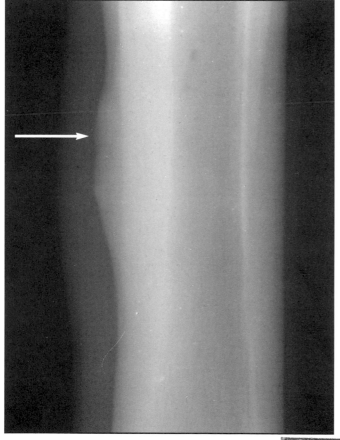

The animal (above) suffered from sore shins and was fired using liquid nitrogen. A radiograph (left) showed that a long-standing fracture of the large metacarpal appeared to have been resolved, but the animal did not subsequently stand training

aggravation of the attachment of the *extensor carpi radialis* tendon at the top of the large metacarpal bone.

Some horses are predisposed to the condition throughout their racing lives. It is observed in young Arab horses that work only on soft ground, and horses ridden on hard, flat beaches may also suffer from it.

Signs

In all cases the shins are very tender when handled, and many affected horses anticipate pain when approached.

Usually no gross abnormality (swelling or enlargement) of the bone is seen, though it will have an obviously convex profile when the shin is bucked.

The condition is suspected when the animal is seen to shorten its stride on ground that does not suit it, and, when the shins are handled after work, the animal will usually exhibit acute pain. Sore shins may affect one or both front limbs (it is unusual in hind limbs, but does occur). Lameness is not always marked, but the animal moves with a short, shuffling gait, possibly because of bilateral pain.

Diagnosis in persistent cases may be helped by radiography to eliminate the presence of detectable metacarpal fractures.

Treatment

While rest is effective (horses do not come in from grass suffering from this condition) the demands of training mean that fit horses are unlikely to be turned out for a condition which appears relatively insignificant and improves well after a few days' rest.

However, it must be appreciated that the injury is a serious one; the periosteum is, in many cases, inflamed and the underlying bone could be fractured.

All sorts of surface treatments are used, and laser and ultrasound therapy are the most effective for relieving the symptoms. While these forms of treatment reduce inflammation and pain, it does not mean the primary problem is resolved. Horses may continue to perform but the healing process may not be completed, and greater injury may result.

In the past, fractures of the cannon have been said to have resulted from treatment of sore shins with ultrasound, but there is no scientific proof to support this. The problem may have arisen from relieving the pain while not fully diagnosing the bony injury. Fracture may simply occur as a natural progression from existing injuries being subjected to further stress.

In recent times there has been interest in the use of liquid nitrogen for this condition, stimulating healing through a form of counter irritation. While early impressions suggest the treatment shows promise it is not yet possible to be sure about it. Many horses have to be turned out before the condition heals fully.

Sesamoiditis

The term sesamoiditis indicates inflammation of the proximal sesamoid bones and/or their ligamentous attachments.

Definition
The proximal sesamoid bones lie one on either side at the back of the fetlock, behind the lower end of the large metacarpal bone, with which they articulate. Each sesamoid is a three-sided pyramid, and moulded to correspond with the hinder end of the large metacarpal bone at its lower end. The posterior surface of each lies beside its fellow to provide a smooth channel which is covered by ligament. At this position the superficial flexor tendon is in the form of a ring through which the deep flexor glides, and the tendons are bound further by the annular (round) ligament of the

Radiograph showing fracture of the proximal sesamoid bone

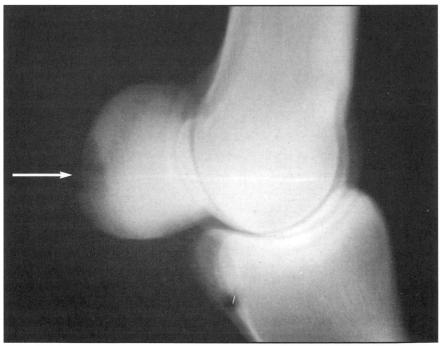

fetlock joint. The sesamoids act together to form a pulley over which the deep flexor tendon runs. A number of very strong ligaments bind the sesamoids into the suspensory apparatus, which increases the surface area of the fetlock joint and helps receive the compression force transmitted downwards from the large metacarpal bone above.

The sesamoids are subjected to a great degree of strain on occasion; this may lead to injury which affects the bones themselves or the ligaments through which they are attached.

Causes

The sesamoid bones may be injured, even fractured, through trauma or as a result of axial forces, and this can lead to considerable swelling which may further complicate movement.

The ligaments attached to the sesamoids may be torn away, bringing with them small pieces of bone, and, because of the dependent anatomy of the region, lameness can become chronic. This is because the ligament ends tend to pull apart and are unable to heal; treatment has to be aimed at counteracting this effect.

Over-extension of the fetlock is a probable cause, resulting in tearing where the ligaments attach to the sesamoids. This effect will be accentuated by any conformation that weakens the joint, and by fatigue.

Signs

An animal is always lame with sesamoid injury. In the immediate aftermath, there will be heat and swelling, though this will tend to reduce with time.

It may not be possible to pinpoint pain to the area manually, and it should be stressed that over-vigorous efforts to do this will only aggravate the condition further.

However, the continued presence of heat is significant, even when all other signs of injury have abated; the area of heat is confined to the back and sides of the fetlock. The condition usually develops as the result of a strain or twist to the joint. It is typical of what might happen when a horse places its foot in a hole.

A concomitant injury to the suspensory ligament may further complicate the picture. Diagnosis needs to be supported by radiography.

Treatment

If lameness is acute the joint is immobilised with a tight supporting bandage. Corrective shoeing, elevating the heels, will help relieve the tension on the sesamoids. This support will need to be kept up for a period of weeks, and during that time laser or ultrasound therapy will usually effect a complete cure.

Sesamoid fractures are also successfully treated by this means, and it is possible to use ultrasound by immersing the leg in water during treatment. The water acts as a coupling medium, allowing the ultrasonic waves to reach the injured area.

Villonodular Synovitis

Though not a very important disease, villonodular synovitis does affect the fetlock and knee joints. Its presence may be suspected where there is fluid distension of the joint and extensive fibrous deposits as a result of concussion. The deposit consists of synovial villi and fibrous nodules.

Ringbone

The term ringbone is used to describe two conditions, similar in nature, which are distinguished by their position on the pastern or at the level of the coronet.

Anatomy of the Pastern

The pastern is the area between the lower end of the fetlock and the foot. It is made up of the first and second phalanges, the latter articulating with the third phalanx and navicular bone within the hoof.

The first phalanx is a long bone (long bones have a central medullary cavity) occupying an oblique position between the lower end of the large metacarpal and the upper end of the second phalanx. The second phalanx is a short bone without a medullary cavity and is therefore solid throughout: it lies partly inside and partly above the upper limit of the wall of the hoof and is the first free limb bone to sustain concussion as the foot hits the ground.

The pastern joint lies between the first and second phalanges and is the least moveable of the phalangeal joints; in the normal standing position it is extended. Excessive dorsiflexion is prevented by the ligaments of the joint and by ligaments on the underside between the first and second phalanges. These latter ligaments thus have considerable importance in bearing weight at the back of the digit and in helping to support the pastern joint.

Definition

Ringbone is an abnormal bony outgrowth affecting the phalanges and their ligamentous attachments. It is described as high or low, depending on whether it occurs at the centre of the pastern or in the region of the coronet respectively. The swelling is due to damage to the periosteum and/or the joint and ligaments involved. If it impinges on a joint, or on a point where a tendon moves over bone, the lameness is more serious.

While the incidence of ringbone has declined, it is still common. It is seen in either fore or hind legs, and can finish an animal's competitive career.

Causes

Occurrence of ringbone is usually related to the uses a horse is put to (e.g. draught work or athleticism). Today, the common cause is trauma (a wrench or twist). Formerly, ringbone tended to occur in the front legs of heavy or aged working horses as a result of concussion (possibly combined with trauma).

Early high ringbone formation (left) *about the pastern joint; and* (right) *feeling for heat over the pastern joint, seat of high ringbone*

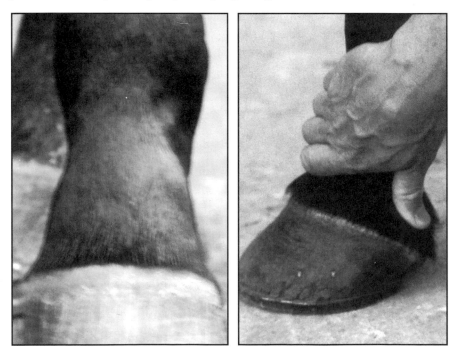

Signs
There is acute reaction with heat and swelling when the injury occurs at exercise. It is vital that any such injury be radiographed in order to locate possible underlying fractures. In more chronic cases, the horse's stride is shortened and the lameness accentuated on rough ground, or when affected animals are turned sharply.

It is easy to distinguish between high and low ringbone by the anatomical position of the swelling. In the mid-pastern area, high ringbone usually surrounds the pastern joint. It should be distinguished from luxation (dislocation) of the joint and it is important to know if the joint itself is involved in the injury (articular ringbone). Low ringbone surrounds the coronary band and usually creates a uniform swelling of the region. The condition may also involve the coffin joint (low articular ringbone).

Treatment
Less serious injuries may be relieved with rest. More serious ones which involve joints are difficult to return to full working soundness, although surgical fusion of the joint may prove effective in a percentage of cases. Some horses are kept in work with the help of phenylbutazone and other non-steroidal anti-inflammatory (NSAID) drugs.

Modern deep treatment with ultrasound, lasers and magnetic field therapy offers great scope for uncomplicated healing in areas of acute bony and ligamentous damage of this nature, but it is important that the problem be approached early and pursued to a satisfactory conclusion. Inevitably the cost of doing this has to be weighed by the animal's owner, as well as the appreciation that not all animals can be returned to full working soundness.

When the injury ends with fusion of two bones through a joint, providing there is no pain on movement, the animal may continue to function adequately but with a somewhat altered gait.

Navicular Disease

While this condition has received a great deal of professional attention in recent times, its position as a cause of lameness is still not properly understood.

Definition
The navicular bone is small and shuttle-shaped, and acts as a fulcrum for the deep flexor tendon before this is attached to the under surface of the

pedal bone. The navicular bone is attached to the wings of the pedal bone by ligaments; it is supported above by ligaments which are attached to its upper border. The navicular bone may become diseased, and the condition can later involve the deep flexor tendon and the bursa that rests between tendon and bone. (A bursa is a synovial sac that reduces friction between moveable parts of the body.)

As the condition progresses, adhesions can form between tendon and bone, and the bone becomes gradually demineralised.

Causes

The causes of the condition are a combination of conformation and concussion arising from work. Contributory causes are poor frog pressure due to bad shoeing, and long toe growth allowing undue strain on the flexor tendons. It may also occur as an upward extension of chronic foot infection.

Various theories have been expounded regarding the causes of this condition, but opinion is returning to the idea that poor foot conformation

Important structures of the lower limb

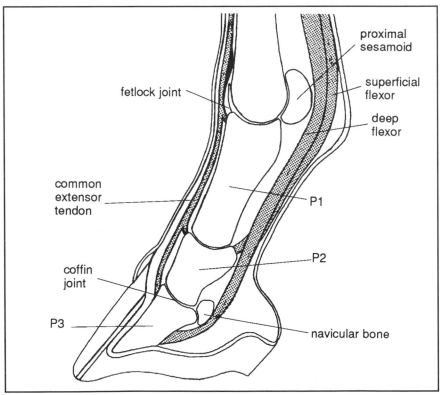

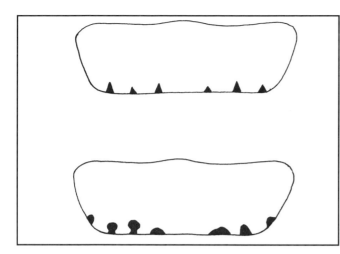

Areas in which bony changes may occur in the navicular bone, as recognised in radiographs. However, such changes are sometimes found in horses which show no lameness

leads to navicular disease, rather than navicular disease leading to conformational changes in the foot.

Signs

The condition has to be considered in all cases of forefoot lameness in horses. However, final confirmation will be dependent on satisfactory radiographic examination. (It should be understood that interpretation of radiographs is known to be controversial and many cases of navicular disease are wrongly diagnosed; it is not always simple to reach a positive decision.)

Navicular disease may be suspected where there is a history of intermittent lameness related to the foot. Often both feet are affected and the stride is short and choppy. At rest, affected feet may be pointed to relieve tension on the painful part. Initial lameness improves as the animal warms up, but may be accentuated when it turns. After rest the symptoms become more pronounced. The shoes of the affected feet are worn at the toe.

Navicular disease is easily confused with other conditions of the lower leg (e.g. sesamoiditis and fetlock joint disease). It is also worth noting that similar gait changes are very often associated with muscular injuries of the shoulder region.

In movement, the foot is placed on the ground toe first in an effort to avoid pressure on the navicular area. If the animal is lunged at the trot the lameness is marked when the affected limb is to the inner side of the circle.

Navicular disease has become the fashionable lameness of our times and many problems are attributed to it incorrectly. A specific diagnosis of the condition necessarily involves the elimination of any other source of abnormailty in the limb.

Treatment
Numerous modern efforts have been made to treat this condition. Warfarin and isoxsuprine are used with some success, although the former treatment is unlikely to have long-term use because of the risks of anticoagulant therapy and the associated tedium of monitoring blood coagaulation times.

The most beneficial approach to bone and ligamentous injuries of the foot is, often, direct forms of deep treatment, using laser or ultrasound. Pain is relieved and animals are kept in work.

Corrective shoeing is utilised to raise the heels and roll the toe. Wedge-shaped pads may be fitted under the shoe to reduce direct concussion to the navicular area. Trimming back the toe encourages more balanced use of the foot and helps promote expansion at the heel.

The use of NSAID drugs may allow animals to be ridden while suffering from this condition but their influence is not curative, although when used in combination with corrective foot care the effect may be more beneficial. Surgery for navicular disease has recently been initiated with some success. Neurectomy may also be carried out, although the risk of other complications increases and it is arguable whether desensitisation is ever really in the long-term interests of the horse.

Pedal Osteitis

Osteitis is inflammation of a bone, in this case the third phalanx (pedal bone).

Definition
The condition often results from jarring on hard ground, which leads to demineralisation or periosteal bone-spur development.

Pedal osteitis is slow to develop and changes may be evident radiographically before the animal is found to be lame.

Causes
Concussion or bruising are common causes, but pedal osteitis may also occur as a sequel to corns, laminitis or punctures of the sole. It is also more common with age because the feet lose shape and texture; the sole flattens thus increasing concussion on the bone. Repeated concussion

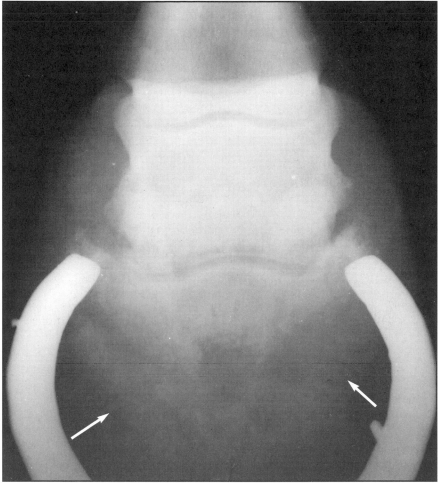

In this radiograph the third phalanx is unclear and there are areas of demineralisation suggestive of pedal osteitis

extending to pedal osteitis was the commonest cause of horses being lost to military service during the two world wars.

Signs
There may be pain on pressure of the sole. The condition usually affects both forefeet which will alter the horse's action: it may tend to shuffle and shorten its stride rather than exhibit overt one-sided lameness. The animal moves more freely on soft surfaces.

Diagnosis is made by radiographic examination when the demineralisation of the bone is clearly defined. The condition must not be confused

with the normal pedal bone variations which are sometimes seen in sound horses. Lameness may not be marked early in the condition but increases with time.

Treatment
As the underlying condition involves demineralisation of bone, this is a process which is unlikely to be reversed. In many cases, anatomical changes which have already occurred in the foot, increasing concussion, are permanent. However, treatment with ultrasound or laser therapy can relieve the symptoms enough for the animal to be kept in work. Radiographic examination shows that this treatment often improves the condition and signs of bone remineralisation are sometimes seen. The affected feet are submerged in water for treatment with ultrasound.

Relief of the symptoms in this condition may be helped by good foot care. This entails careful balancing of the feet and ensuring that the shoes do not bear on sensitive tissues. The effects of concussion may be reduced by leather or plastic pads. In some cases, plastic shoes may provide immediate relief.

Sidebone

Sidebone arises when the lateral cartilages of the foot are converted into bone (ossified).

Definition
When functioning normally these cartilages, which attach to the wings of the pedal bone, are part of the shock-absorbing system of the foot. When they become bony, through the effects of concussion or direct injury, this facility is lost.

The condition is most common in heavy and plain-bred horses.

Causes
Concussion is the usual cause of sidebone, which was most commonly seen in working horses that drew heavy loads in city streets. In these animals, treads were also a common cause (treads are injuries to the coronet inflicted by the horse's opposite foot, or, in the case of harness horses, by the adjacent horse).

Ossification of the cartilages also occurs occasionally in young horses and may represent a physiological response to the combined influences of development and concussion.

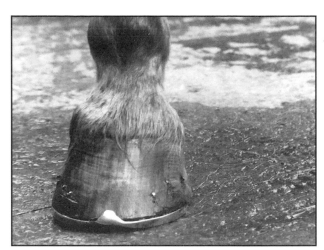

Sidebones account for the prominence of the coronet (left), *especially in the lateral view* (centre) *and as indicated by the fingers on the lateral cartilage* (below)

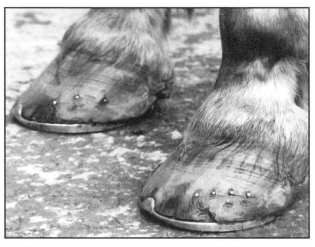

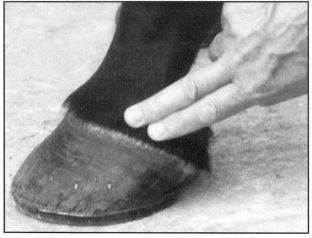

Signs

Lameness is not a common feature except in the early stages of sidebone, while the process of ossification is taking place. However, persistent lameness can occur with fully developed sidebones due to pressure on the wall of the foot from within.

The hardened cartilages are felt at the junction of hair and hoof in the region of the quarter of the foot.

Radiographs may help in confirming the diagnosis.

Treatment

When lameness is negligible or absent the condition is not normally treated. Once the cartilage has become ossifed, lameness is uncommon.

Maintaining proper foot care ensures correct balance and a level foot/ground plane. Grooving of the feet sometimes helps to relieve pressure over the ossified cartilages where lameness exists.

Bone Spavin

The term spavin is used to describe diseases of the hock joint.

Anatomy

The hock joint is a complex structure consisting of the six small tarsal bones and their articulation with the tibia above, with each other, and with the large metatarsal bone below. There are, therefore, four main articulations involved, namely, the tibiotarsal, the proximal and distal intertarsal, and the tarsometatarsal joints.

The bones of the hock are the calcaneus (forming the point of the hock), the talus (articulating with the tibia) and two rows of smaller bones comprising the central tarsal, the fourth tarsal, the third tarsal and the fused first and second tarsal bones.

Definition

Bone spavin is the term used to describe a bony enlargement on the inner side of the hock due to inflammation of joints, bone and ligaments in the area. It can involve the upper end of the cannon bone and the bones and joints of the hock nearby. The result may be DJD leading to obliteration of the affected joints (most commonly the distal intertarsal and tarsometatarsal joints) and fusion of the affected bones.

Causes
The condition is related to poor hock conformation, coupled with concussive injury to the area. When formed, bone spavin is readily recognised at the junction of the lower end of the hock and beginning of the cannon bone on the inner side of the leg. However, in early cases there may be little or no abnormal bone growth.

Sickle hocks and cow hocks are said to lead to spavin, but it is the influence of these types of conformation on axial forces that probably concentrates injury in this area.

Signs
Lameness is most pronounced when trotting from standing, or when the horse first pulls out; the effects of lameness diminish with exercise.

In the early stages of the condition, the animal may become lame following a period of rest after fast work (without any evident swelling). The action of the affected limb may be altered, with wear on the outside of the shoe. Flexion of the joint may be reduced and the horse will then track short on the affected side. There is a tendency for the shoe on the affected side to be worn at the toe, but this can also occur as a result of other sources of lameness.

Spavin is suggested by the typical swelling on the inside of the hock. Even in early cases where the bone has not increased in size, heat is usually marked over the site.

Picking the leg up and flexing the hock for anything longer than thirty seconds is the basis of the 'spavin test'. However, it is important to remember that this process automatically also flexes the stifle, and may flex the fetlock and lower limb joints. The test is not specific and other sources of lameness will be accentuated through the same process. When the limb is released the horse is trotted away and lameness is marked if the horse has spavin.

The condition is confirmed radiographically.

Bone spavin usually develops as a single-leg lameness but can subsequently occur in the other limb. There can also be parallel spavin development in both limbs at the same time.

Treatment
Bone spavin does not respond well to treatment and tends to be progressive once developed. Rest and other treatments may well alleviate the signs but if the horse is returned to full work lameness often recurs. In a percentage of cases movement of the affected joint may be obliterated by new bone growth and the animal may then become functionally sound.

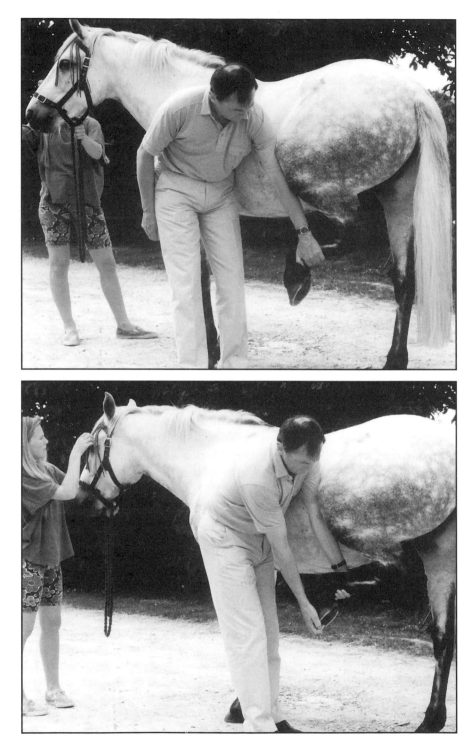

OPPOSITE PAGE: *Flexing the hind limb is the basis of the spavin test. Flexing the hock* (above) *without flexing the lower limb joints; and* (below) *flexing the lower limb joints as well. Note that the stifle is also being flexed, the weight-bearing limb is taking added weight and the horse's back is also affected*

This process may be fostered by keeping the animal in work with the help of phenylbutazone.

Surgery for the condition is quite effective, offering about a 60 per cent chance of a full return to work after a recovery period of six to twelve months. Its goal is to promote joint fusion and thereby alleviate pain.

Corrective shoeing is aimed at balancing the foot when it lands on the ground. This may be achieved by altering the breakover (the point in the stride at which the foot leaves the ground) through the application of a stud or trailer (a backward extension) on the outer branch of the shoe.

In some cases the horse remains technically unsound but is able to continue work.

Types of Spavin

1)   Occult, or blind, spavin is spavin lameness with no bony swelling.
2)   Jack spavin is a large bone spavin.
3)   High spavin, located higher on the hock than normal bone spavin.
4)   Bog spavin is a chronic swelling of the hock joint itself with soft swelling on the front and back of the hock.

Subchondral Bone Cysts

Subchondral means 'beneath cartilage' and refers to the cartilage involved in joint formation in the present context.

Definition
Subchondral bone cysts are cavities that develop in the substance of long bones, close to a joint, very often at the point of maximum weight bearing. They may or may not communicate with the joint and may contain synovial fluid. These cysts occur in many different situations but are most common in the lower end of the femur. They occur in both young and older horses.

Causes
The position of the cyst suggests that axial forces play a part in causing them. There may also be a nutritional influence.

Signs

Lameness is variable in this condition, depending mostly on whether or not the cyst comes in contact with a joint; in which case lameness can be acute and persistent. There may be no external signs of joint swelling.

Diagnosis depends on complete examination of the lame limb and exclusion of other sources of lameness. The bone cyst is located by radiographic examination.

Treatment

It is possible that a percentage of cases will resolve with rest. However, this is less likely where there is joint involvement and surgery is required in these cases to excavate the cyst and promote repair.

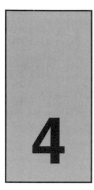

4 | The Foot

The foot is often said to be the most common source of lameness in horses today, but with the exception of infection and bruising (both of which are often related to shoeing) lameness originating in this complex structure is comparable to that in the fetlock or knee. It is probably considerably less common than lameness originating from the muscular system and spinal structures of competing horses (in which foot care is fully understood and less likely to be neglected than in non-competing animals). Nevertheless, foot lameness is of suffecent importance to warrant treatment as a separate entity.

It is imperative that examinations for lameness in any limb involve methodical examination of the whole limb starting with the comprehensive examination of the foot.

Anatomy of the Foot

The parts of the foot are divided thus:

a) The hoof and other external structures (insensitive foot, part of the epidermis).

b) The sensitive foot (derived from the dermis, existing between horn and bone).

c) The bones and cartilages of the foot.

d) The coffin joint.

The hoof is composed of modified skin similar to the horns and claws of other animals and is made up of the following structures.

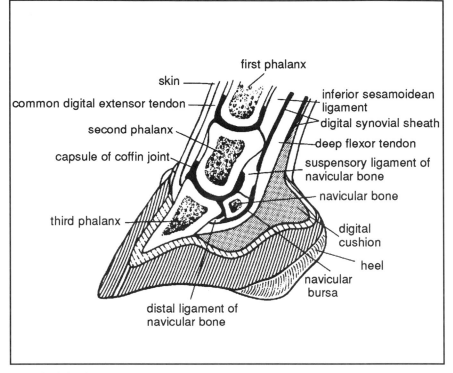

Detail of the foot

The Insensitive Foot

The insensitive foot is comprised of the wall, the sole, the frog and the bars.

The Wall

This is the part which can be seen when the foot is on the ground. It is composed of dense horn (water content 25 per cent) on the inner surface of which are the insensitive laminae, and it is arbitrarily divided into toe, quarters and heels.

The wall is developed by a downward growth of horn secreted by cells of the coronary band (the coronary cushion), a ring of modified skin. Above the coronary band is a similar but smaller cushion, the perioplic ring. This secretes a layer of waterproof varnish over the wall to prevent loss of moisture and the resultant hoof shrinkage. The rate of growth from the coronary band permits the complete replacement of the horny wall in a period of 8-10 months.

When the rate of growth is irregular, alternating ridges and circular depressions encircle the wall; this can be influenced by diet. When horn growth is accelerated, as when out on spring grass, raised grass-rings are produced. When horses rough it in winter, circular depressions may appear later. Deeper and wider circular grooves follow an attack of laminitis.

The Sole

The sole (water content 33 per cent) constitutes the greater part of the ground surface of the hoof. It is crescent-shaped and arched in relation to the ground, and provides protection for the foot, acting as a shock-absorber.

In the clean, unshod foot the line of union between wall and sole is quite visible just inside the inner margin of the wall and is known as the white line. At the hinder part of the sole it can be seen to turn inwards and forwards to form an inner lining to the bars. When nailing on a shoe it is important that the nail neither punctures this division between horny and sensitive parts, nor presses unduly on it to cause nail-binding. It is at the white line that separation occurs in seedy toe.

The Frog

This is a wedge-shaped structure interposed between the bars. It is made up of spongy horn which consists of about 50 per cent water. Its function is to absorb concussion and assist circulation to the structures of the foot.

The frog extends considerably below the level of the sole and comes into contact with the ground during normal movement.

In a correctly shod foot the weight of the body falls upon the wall, bars and frog when the horse is in motion. When only the wall receives weight, the buffering effect of the fibrous cushion, which overlies the frog, is lost. The result is greater strain on higher structures of the leg, such as the fetlock, cannon and tendons, and limb circulation also suffers.

The Bars

At the heel, the horny wall bends forwards and inwards to meet the front angle of the frog. The inturned wall forms an upright partition of horn and this, together with the upright wall of the heel, constitutes the bar of the foot.

The purpose of the bar is to take additional weight upon the heel. Except during the slow walk, when the foot lands virtually level, horses place their feet with the heel first, then the frog, and finally the toe, as the body travels over the area occupied by the foot. Each time this happens the frog should take the weight, force the angle of the bars open, and prevent the heels from caving in and contracting.

The Sensitive Foot

The sensitive foot is comprised of the coronary band, the corium of the foot and perioplic ring.

The Coronary Band or Cushion

This encircles the coronet from one bulb of heel to the other, and is situated at the junction of the wall and skin. It produces horn cells for the growth of the hoof.

The Corium of the Foot

The laminar corium covers the outer surface of the pedal bone. (The corium is the fibrous inner layer of the skin just beneath the epidermis.) It is provided with about 600 leaf-like sensitive laminae, which interlock with the insensitive laminae of the hoof wall and hold the pedal bone in position. Covering the lower surface of the pedal bone is the corium of the sole (sensitive sole), and covering the undersurface of the digital cushion is the corium of the frog (sensitive frog). These components of the corium are continuous with one another and are well supplied with blood vessels and nerves. They provide nourishment for the production of the horny parts of the wall, sole and frog.

Lying between the two lateral cartilages is a mass of fibrous elastic tissue, the digital (pedal or plantar) cushion, situated between the undersurface of the pedal bone and frog. It has a poor blood supply and is not very sensitive. This pad is moulded over the inner face of the horny frog and its purpose is to act as a buffer and lessen concussion when the foot meets the ground. It extends back to the bulbs of the heel and out to the lateral cartilages under the walls of the hoof.

The Perioplic Ring

Situated around the hoof, above the coronary band, the perioplic ring secretes a layer of waterproof varnish which covers the wall. Its purpose is to prevent moisture loss and accompanying shrinkage of the hoof and splitting of the wall.

The Bones of the Foot and Cartilages

Although part of the second phalanx is included in the foot, our main concern here is with the third phalanx and the distal sesamoid (navicular) bone.

The Third Phalanx
The third phalanx (pedal or coffin bone) is the terminal bone of the limb and resembles the hoof in shape, but is very much smaller and occupies only a minor portion of the cavity within the hoof. The deep flexor tendon is attached to it below and behind. Between the deep flexor and the upper part of the hind face of the bone is the navicular bone. There is a bursa interposed between these.

The highest point of the third phalanx is the extensor process at the front. This gives attachment to the tendon of the common digital extensor which advances the foot and extends the fetlock and knee joints.

The articular surface is moulded to that of the lower end of the second phalanx, and also carries a facet behind which articulates with the navicular bone.

Cartilages of the Foot
The angles of the third phalanx on either side give support to the cartilages of the foot. On their inner aspect the cartilages meet the digital cushion and in front they afford protection to the coffin joint. The upper border of each cartilage is thin and flexible and can be moved sideways with the fingers just above the coronary band. They bulge outwards every time weight falls on the heel and frog.

The cartilages are attached to the bony structures of the foot by a number of ligaments. They are hyaline (translucent with no fibres) in the young (reflected in their pliability) but turn to fibrocartilage in the adult (gaining the consistency of bone).

The Coffin Joint

The coffin joint lies within the hoof and is formed between the second and third phalanges and the navicular bone; it exhibits a great degree of movement. In the normal standing position the joint is extended; over-extension being limited by a suspensory apparatus and the deep flexor tendon behind.

Conditions of the Foot

The conditions listed here are additions to those already described earlier for concussive lameness. Other conditions of foot lameness, such as laminitis, are listed separately according to cause.

Contraction

It is important to the effective functioning of the foot that the whole structure be fully expanded and properly formed. Anatomical changes from the normal may be tolerated but are a common cause, or effect, of disease.

Definition
Contraction of the foot is usually unilateral. The affected foot is smaller than its partner and the difference is, therefore, easily recognised. The foot is shrunken and the walls upright and boxy.

Sole of foot (right) *with a contracted frog; foot with degenerated frog* (below, *right), associated with a keratoma; shoeing a normal foot* (below) *which has a well-developed frog*

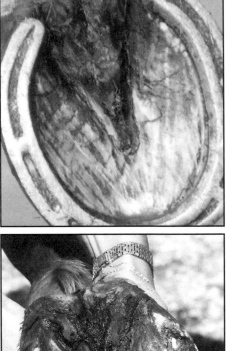

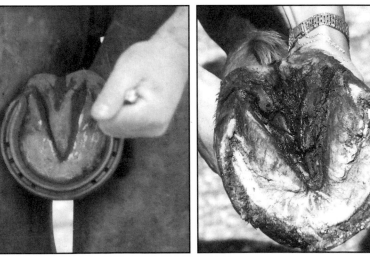

Bilateral contraction can also occur but there is still little difficulty in recognising the signs. The angle of the walls, shrinking of the frog and lack of foot expansion are all typical.

It may happen in any foot, though it is more common in front.

Causes
The heels contract owing to lack of frog pressure. This happens either because of faulty shoeing or when the wall at the heel is allowed to grow too long. It can also happen with any chronic lameness in which the heel is not brought into contact with the ground. Contraction at the heel is easily identified and may precede overall contraction of the foot. When established the problem may take some time to correct.

Signs
On examination, the frog will be high and have a shrunken appearance. Where only one foot is affected, its size in comparison to the other is notably smaller. The hoof may have a boxy and upright appearance, and the wall may be dry owing to the influence of contraction on the coronary band.

There are various grades of this condition depending on the length of time frog pressure has been lost. Contraction is commonly seen in young foals but can quickly be reversed with good foot care.

Treatment
The aim is to restore frog pressure. The heels are pared down to bring the frog into closer contact with the ground. A special shoe with a pad or bar may be worn to assist this purpose.

Corns

Corns in the horse differ from the human condition so named in that they result from direct pressure on sensitive tissues, resulting in bleeding, not thickening of skin.

Definition
A corn is a bruise of the sensitive foot at the angle between the wall and bar at the heel. It is more common in forefeet where it may occur at either angle.

Causes
The normal cause is the shoe bearing directly on the sole at the seat of

The shaded area is commonly affected by bruising. The spots represent the seat of corn

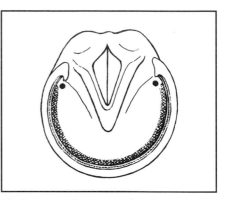

corn. This may result when shoes are left on too long, or if a shoe moves inward from the wall. Alternatively, a stone may wedge under the branch of a shoe, causing the same problem. A less common cause is the development of bony spurs on the wings, or angles, of the pedal bone. These result from concussion and can create a persistent problem.

Horses differ in their tendency to corns. A great deal depends on the shape of the foot and texture of the horn. Flat feet with soft soles create an evident problem which may be difficult to overcome. In some such cases it may not be possible to apply conventional shoes.

Signs

During early corn development, bruising may be seen and blood become evident beneath the pared surface of the sole at the heel. Later the sole takes on a yellowish appearance and superficial tissues degenerate.

There are varying degrees of lameness depending on the hardness of the ground. There may be heat in the region of the heels, and the blood vessels on the affected side of the leg may be tense and pulsing. When moving, the animal tries to avoid bearing weight on the affected part, but will usually trot more soundly on a soft surface. Where the corn leads to infection of the sensitive foot, lameness will be marked.

The shoe will need to be removed to expose the corn when the animal will flinch on application of pressure to the part. The damaged tissue can be seen quite clearly at the seat of corn.

Treatment

The damaged tissue is pared back and, if infection has gone to the sensitive foot, drainage is established. Poultices are then applied to draw off accumulated matter, and antibiotics may be needed in obstinate cases.

A seated-out shoe should be fitted to avoid further pressure on the site. Care needs to be taken with future shoeing because the condition may recur. In some cases a three-quarter shoe will be necessary to allow the damaged tissue to grow back.

Prevention of tetanus is wise in all cases of infection of the foot.

Bruised Sole

Bruising of the feet is a regular problem in shod horses. It is less common in animals reared in the wild.

Definition
Bruising of the sole is seen when the superficial layers of horn are pared back and the presence of blood is identified in the underlying tissues. It results from external pressure on sensitive tissues.

Causes
The sole is bruised as a result of the horse treading on stones (or other foreign objects), or commonly results from shoe pressure on the sensitive sole. The latter cause may occur because the sole has dropped, leaving the farrier with little room in which to place the shoe. Neglect, by not removing shoes when needed or when a shoe loosens and moves inwardly in the course of normal riding, is also a cause.

Signs
Bruising is quite easily identified when the surface of the horn is pared back with a hoof knife over the damaged area. Traces of blood will be seen (most commonly under the bearing surface of the shoe). Lameness is generally pronounced. Pain is usually evinced if the injured area is subjected to pressure, even with a thumb.

Treatment
The horse may be reshod as long as the shoe does not bear on the bruised region. Alternatively the animal may need to be rested until the pain has gone and the injured tissues have repaired.

Severe bruising of the sole may be associated with injury to the pedal bone and radiography may be necessary to eliminate this possibility.

Various forms of physiotherapy prove beneficial in relieving the symptoms after bruising. Both ultrasound and laser therapy are effective in reducing inflammation and returning horses to work quickly.

Dropped Sole
Changes in the shape of the feet occur commonly with age. Alterations in

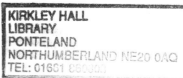

the relationship of the sole with the ground are accordingly a serious feature of this.

Definition
Dropped sole exists when the ground surface of the foot loses its natural concavity and the sensitive tissues of the sole become exposed to injury through direct trauma. It is a natural anatomical defect in some lines of horses.

Causes
The condition is a common sequel to laminitis, but occurs as a natural part of the ageing process in many horses. It can also result from careless foot trimming which excessively shortens the hoof walls and allows the sole to lose support.

In isolated cases, improper balancing of the foot may cause the sole to collapse on one side. Correction may then result in a completely flattened foot.

Signs
The shape of the sole changes over a period of time. It assumes a position that is perpendicular to the wall and makes it difficult for the farrier to apply shoes without risk of bruising. The problem is easily recognised with basic understanding of normal foot conformation.

Treatment
In some cases, when dropped sole arises in young animals, regular trimming may restore the natural contour of the sole.

Where the condition is more advanced, leather or plastic pads may help to prevent bruising, although in advanced cases this may not work. Plastic shoes are sometimes effective in these cases because of their basic design which tends to make maximum use of the weight-bearing capacity of the wall.

It is critical that the shoe should not bear on the sensitive structures of the sole at any point; this may be achieved with the help of seated-out shoes. However, this is sometimes impossible to achieve and the animal's subsequent career is almost inevitably curtailed.

When the shape of the sole has changed owing to improper balancing, it is vital that this be corrected at as early a stage as possible. In these cases it is vital to aim at restoring the natural shape of the sole as well as correcting foot balance. Failure to do so is certain to shorten the active life of the animal.

Seedy Toe

An alternative name used for this condition is 'hollow wall', a term which describes the sound achieved by tapping an affected foot with an instrument like a hammer.

Definition
With this condition the wall of the foot separates from the sole at the white line. The space thus formed is filled with a soft crumbling horn, and this varies in quantity with the degree of separation.

Causes
The condition is sometimes a sequel to chronic laminitis, and may allow infection into the foot. It may also result from bruising of the toe or excessive clip pressure.

Signs
Seedy toe becomes evident at shoeing. It does not usually produce lameness, except in the presence of infection. The front wall of the foot may be curled forward and exposed to damage in movement, and the horn may be brittle and dry.

Treatment
The dead horn is taken out and prevention of infection can be aided by packing with tow impregnated with a mild antiseptic (a combination of eucalyptus and iodoform is popular) or wound powder. Attention should also be given to the diet to ensure proper horn growth.

The defect will grow out given time, and it is wise to ensure that the

How the wall and sole (left) *separate at the white line in seedy toe. It is possible for this reaction to extend up as far as the coronet, in the area (*shaded, right*) usually affected*

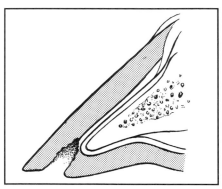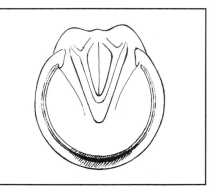

wall at the toe is trimmed back in such a way that it does not become further injured in movement.

Sandcrack

The hoof is a structure similar in nature to the human fingernail. Breaks in its integrity are commonly found.

Definition
Sandcrack describes any break in the hoof wall between ground surface and coronet, running variable distances between these two limits. They may be partial or complete, penetrating through the full thickness of the wall at times. They may occur in any foot and are seen at the toe, quarter or heel.

Extensive sandcrack with healed coronary wound. Such a wound will take a long time to heal unaided. This animal is functionally sound

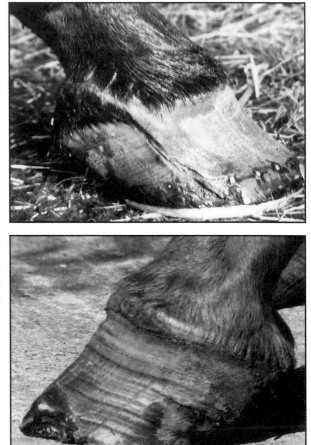

Transverse crack in forefoot with keratoma. Intermittent lameness was a feature of this case

Causes

Sandcracks are caused by injury, or defects in growth at the coronary band; they also occur through neglect or as a result of poor nutrition. Lameness is evident in serious cases.

Horses coming in from grass will invariably have cracks (grasscracks) if the ground is dry and hard and the feet have not been trimmed regularly. These will travel part way up the wall and cause little trouble when shod. However, if the crack opens on contact with the ground, lameness is likely to occur.

Signs

Sandcracks are easily recognisable, but it is important to determine the cause and extent of a crack. If caused by damage to the coronary band, treatment will have to be aimed at protecting the foot and encouraging growth from this area.

Treatment

Where the crack does not extend up the whole length of the wall from the ground, a groove or pattern burned into the top will immobilise it and facilitate healing. A shoe clip may be used for the same purpose. Should the crack reach the bottom of the wall it is trimmed back so that the break does not come in contact with the shoe or ground. The horn may also be grooved to limit the downward extension of cracks commencing at the coronet. Clips or wire sutures may be used to achieve the same end.

Some deep cracks are filled with resinous bonding compounds to prevent the sensitive tissues from being damaged subsequent to movement of the crack.

Where it is necessary to promote horn growth the hoof is dressed daily in hoof oil and the horse is given mineral mixes which provide the essential nutrients needed.

Coronary band injuries respond well to ultrasound and laser therapy, both of which help to promote natural growth of tissues.

Foot Infections

Probably the most common cause of foot lameness, infection is always routinely checked for in any lame limb.

Definition

Infections of the foot occur as a consequence of penetrating injuries. The infection builds up within the foot confines, and accumulated discharges often follow the line of least resistance and break out at the coronet or heel.

Causes

Infections may occur owing to upward migration of grit or gravel through the horn; they may also enter through shoe-nail tracks when these penetrate the white line. Infection also occurs as an upward development from corns or, frequently, because of penetration by foreign bodies such as spikes, nails, or even thorns though these are likely to penetrate the frog.

Signs

Foot infections may be presented as a chronic development or may appear as a cause of acute lameness. The build-up of infectious material within the foot is (evidently) painful and immediate relief is noted on its release.

It is important to distinguish infection from physical injuries to the foot (such as bruises and corns), and also fractures of the pedal and navicular bones.

Treatment

Shoes must first be removed (in these cases). The source of primary infection can usually be limited by the vet or farrier to a restricted area, by judicious examination with a hoof knife and with pressure applied by a hoof tester.

It is then often possible to locate the track and follow it through to the sensitive tissues and allow pus to escape. (Each suspected track should be pursued until healthy tissue is found, at which point the searching must stop. There is no need to draw blood, which is only an indication that the search has already gone too far. The infected track will generally release infected material and no healthy tissue will be seen right through to the point of pus release.)

Many foot infections recover after this simple procedure. However, many cases are more difficult to treat and it may be necessary to apply poultices to help draw off all accumulated infection. In some cases the location is difficult to identify and little or no pus may be found.

Antibiotics are needed only in persistent cases, but it is always wise to ensure cover for tetanus.

More obstinate cases may require surgical intervention to promote adequate drainage.

Radiographs may need to be taken to eliminate the possibility of fractures or other foot conditions.

Thrush and Canker

These are both conditions that often arise through management errors. They should therefore be avoidable.

Definition
Thrush is a degenerative condition of the frog in which there is tissue decay, denoted by a foul smell, and varying degrees of infection. Canker is a similar type of condition but more serious in its effects. It is marked by underrunning of the sole and frog (i.e. when infection effectively separates superficial and deep layers of the foot). In advanced cases, areas of the sensitive sole may be exposed.

Causes
Thrush and canker occur owing to dirty, wet underfoot conditions. They normally reflect poor standards of stable management which force animals to stand in rank and fetid bedding. These conditions may occur in either fore or hind feet and may be present in more than one foot at the same time.

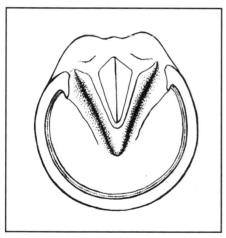

The areas (dappled) *between the frog and the bar of the foot, the lateral sulci, are the most common site of thrush*

Signs
With thrush, the cleft of the frog is moist and evil smelling, and it is not unusual for the problem to extend through to the sensitive foot and set up infection within.

The frog itself may be undermined and the lateral grooves (sulci) between frog and horn found to be deeper than normal. A black discharge may be present.

Diagnosis is based on the condition of the frog, the presence of excessive moisture, undermining, and the characteristic evil smell.

With canker, a heavy, evil-smelling discharge may come from infected tissues, but it is equally possible that there may be no smell. The horn may be decayed, of a soft, oily texture, and easily separated to expose the sensitive tissues. The whole foot, up to the coronary band, may be involved.

Both conditions may exist without lameness in the early stages, but lameness is almost certain as the conditions develop.

Diagnosis is based on examination of the foot and exposure of the dead and rotting tissues.

Treatment

For thrush, the affected area of the frog should be opened out and exposed to the air. The foot should be immersed in a solution of 5 per cent copper sulphate, or formalin. Where there is infection of the sensitive foot, drainage must be established where possible. Antibiotics (or antifungal drugs) are indicated in severe cases.

All diseased areas are pared away in canker and infection limited by use of antiseptic and antibiotic packs. The sensitive areas must be protected until healing and new horn growth occurs, and this can take months to achieve.

Canker may be resistant to treatment, recurrence being common if all infected tissue is not removed.

Prevention

These problems are prevented by careful attention to stable and foot hygiene. Feet should be picked out regularly and dressed with a suitable hoof dressing. Underfoot conditions need to be kept dry and clean.

Quittor

The extension of foot infections may involve deeper anatomical structures. Such a condition is quittor.

Definition

Persistent infections involving the lateral cartilages are described as quittor. Discharge may occur periodically in some cases.

Causes

Quittor usually results from a foot infection that gains access to a lateral cartilage causing necrosis of areas of this structure. It is marked by an

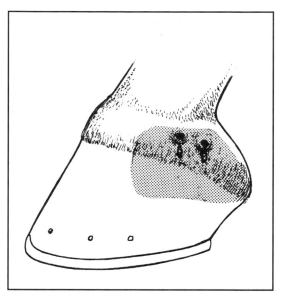

Quittor involves infection of the lateral cartilages which may lead to the appearance of disch(ar)ing tracts at the coronet

open sinus (or sinuses) at the coronary band that extrude purulent material to the outside.

Signs
The condition is chronic in nature and is easily identified by its situation over the affected cartilage.

Treatment
While conservative therapy, involving poultices, drainage and antibiotics may occasionally prove successful, many cases of quittor do not clear up without surgical intervention. This necessitates excavation of the infected site and the establishment of effective drainage.

Keratoma

Tumours of the foot are not that common, but they do occur and are important to recognise for diagnostic reasons.

Definition
A keratoma is a benign tumour that grows usually in the front of the foot between the wall and the pedal bone.

Causes
Keratoma may occur as a sequel to infection or trauma. But the cause is

A left foreleg keratoma causing distortion of the front wall, disturbance of the coronet and horn growth defects

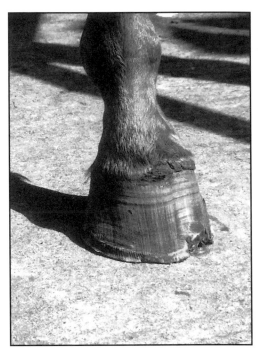

not fully understood and the possibility exists that the condition could result from a number of factors, e.g. a combination of injury, concussion and infection.

Signs

The presence of a keratoma may be suspected when there is a deformity of the front wall of the foot with a history of chronic repeated discharge of pus at the coronary band.

Lameness is common when infection is building up and less when it is released. Affected horses may lead relatively normal existences although periods of lameness intervene. The condition is least painful on soft ground.

Radiographs will be needed to confirm the diagnosis.

Treatment

While some horses suffering from this condition may be kept virtually sound by constant attention to accompanying infections, radical surgery, opening the hoof wall and removing the tumour, is necessary to effect a full cure.

The severity of the symptoms will depend on the size of the growth, its influence on surrounding tissues and the degree of pain it causes. Thus, milder cases may be manageable without surgery, while more severe cases will not. After surgery the horse will be out of action for some time because the removed horn will take 8-10 months to grow back, and the tumour can recur.

Buttress Foot

Physical injuries to the front of the foot and its underlying structures may lead to the condition known as buttress foot.

Definition
This condition is diagnosed where there is localised swelling at the front of the coronet immediately above the pyramidal process of the third phalanx.

Causes
Buttress foot occurs as a consequence of fracture or periostitis of the pyramidal process, and involves the attachment of the digital extensor tendon to this process of the bone.

Signs
The condition is similar to low ringbone except that it is restricted to the extensor process; the coffin joint is not usually affected.

Swelling is seen at the front of the coronet and there is abnormal hoof growth in the same region due to pressure on the coronary band.

Treatment
It is possible that shoeing with a full roller-motion shoe will encourage movement. A roller-motion shoe has a rounded ground surface that allows

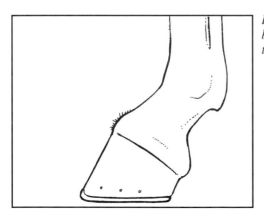

Buttress foot is related to bony changes at the front of the coronet

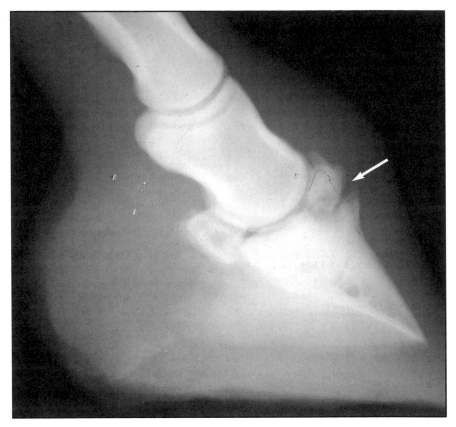

Fracture of the pyramidal process of the third phalanx. This is the underlying lesion in buttress foot

adjustment at the point of breakover. The condition, however, which is not commonly seen today, does not lend itself to conventional treatments, including surgery.

Club Foot

Foot deformities that limit use are uncommon in the horse. The hereditary occurrence of such conditions is rare and animals suffering this condition are unlikely to be bred from.

Definition
The condition is similar to, but more advanced than, contracted foot. The foot is shrunken, upright, and there is apparent contraction of the deep

flexor tendon. This contraction may ensue from a relative disproportion in length between bone and tendon during active phases of growth. Club foot can be unilateral or bilateral.

Causes
Club foot occurs as a consequence of any disease which results in tendon contraction and improper use of the affected foot. The underlying cause may be nutritional in younger animals exhibiting disproportionate bone and tendon growth.

Signs
The foot is shrunken and upright, giving it a contracted, boxy appearance. The animal will walk on the toe and may have difficulty placing the heel on the ground.

Treatment
Where the condition occurs bilaterally in foals, correction of the diet is necessary and surgical interference (the inferior check ligament is sectioned) may be required to relieve the effect of tendon contraction. Where surgery is not carried out, the heels are raised to prevent further aggravation of the tendons. Later, when normal tendon/bone conformation is restored, the feet may need to be trimmed to correct the boxy development, shortening the heels as much as possible to encourage expansion and restore frog use.

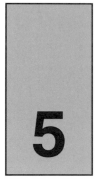

5 Constitutional and Developmental Lameness

In this chapter we are concerned with those lamenesses which relate to the constitutional make up of an animal and which develop due to a number of factors concerning the animal's heredity and environment.

Laminitis

Though more common in ponies than in larger breeds of horse, laminitis is one of the major causes of lameness seen. Its occurrence is ubiquitous and the wastage of animals as a result of laminitis is high. This is expressed in death (perhaps for humane reasons), loss of use and shortened working life.

Although the principle signs of laminitis are confined to the feet, the condition is not a primary foot disease in most cases, because the precipitating cause may exist in remote regions, like the bowel, or the uterus in the mare.

However, laminitis was known in earlier times as 'fever of the feet', recognising the most common symptoms seen - namely heat and pain - in the feet. Varying numbers of feet may be affected.

Diagnosis

The conditions that lead to laminitis are fairly standard.
1)   Excessive intake of rich grass in small, fat ponies.
2)   As a sequel to grain overload (e.g. when an animal breaks into a grain store and gorges itself).

3)   As a sequel to retained afterbirth in the mare.

4)   As a complication of diarrhoea or other digestive abnormalities.

5)   Following the consumption of large amounts of cold water after exercise. It is suggested that the consumption of water does not precipitate the condition, although it may permit the changes in the bowel that do.

6)   As a sequel to bad shoeing when shoes are placed too tightly and the nails impinge on the sensitive tissues of the foot.

7)   When excess weight bearing imposes stress on a single foot (usually a forefoot) because of lameness in its fellow limb.

8)   As a consequence of excessive concussion.

9)   Laminitis may also result from the use of corticosteroids.

10)   Stress is named as a common factor (e.g. travel). However, it is not beyond imagination that the influence here could be disturbed digestion with toxin production, in common with other digestive forms of the disease.

It can be seen from the above that the causes of laminitis lie within a few parameters, mainly toxic and mechanical, and it is possible that all precipitating causes of the condition can be reduced to these basic headings. However, as yet, the pathological cause of laminitis is not fully understood, although knowledge in veterinary science has considerably widened in recent years.

The changes which are recognised in toxic laminitis relate to an interference with normal blood circulation through the laminar corium of the foot. There are two contradictory events here: on the one hand there is ischaemia (deficiency of blood) to the laminae; on the other there is an increase of blood to other structures of the foot. The reason these two events occur at the same time is due to an external influence on local vessels, causing constriction of vessels supplying the laminae (and thus restricted blood flow). Blood is effectively shunted from the arteries to the veins without perfusing the deprived area. Inevitably, the longer this lasts the greater damage that is done to the vessels involved and consequently to the laminae, and the more serious the symptoms that appear.

The pain felt is due to the pathological reaction in the laminae, which are deprived of oxygen and nutrients. The consequence of this deprivation, if it lasts for any length of time, is separation of the sensitive and insensitive laminae, and hence the attachment that exists between the third phalanx and hoof wall. Detachment begins at the front of the foot and is accompanied by a rotation of the bone downwards. This process is aided by the weight of the animal bearing down from above as well as the pull

Cross-section of horse's foot with detail (insert) of sensitive (white) and insensitive (black) laminae

of the deep flexor tendon attached to the rear. The effect is compounded by the effusion of blood and serum into space so created.

From here the condition is progressive and the downward movement of the bone results in dropping of the sole and possible penetration through the horn of the tip of the bone itself.

Signs
While heat is not a constant feature of the condition it is common enough to have an important diagnostic significance. Its presence in many horses without advanced symptoms of the disease indicates that there are varying grades of the condition and that these symptoms are often reversed without major clinical changes developing.

Heat is felt by hand in the region of the coronary band and over the wall of the hoof.

The condition is divided into acute and chronic forms. The acute form appears suddenly and the animal is unable to move without great pain. If the forelegs alone are affected the animal gets its hind feet under its body to relieve the weight on the forelegs. This stance may confuse an owner into thinking there is a problem in the back. If the horse is made to turn, it will appear that the forelegs are being lifted off the ground after which the feet are put down gently, heels first. The horse may be sweating and have a rise in temperature. As a general rule, heat is felt in the affected feet.

Chronic cases occur as an after-effect of acute attacks. The level of pain is less, but heat is still detectable in the foot and the animal suffers at all gaits. It bears weight on its heels and there is a gradual change in the shape of the feet. The toe elongates and turns upwards and the heel and pastern respond accordingly. The sole flattens and the tip of the pedal bone may occasionally penetrate through.

The signs of laminitis are dependent on varying degrees of pain in one or more feet. There are also changes in the substance of the foot itself, ranging from mere heat detected by hand, and pain (noticeable in movement), to the gross changes already mentioned, i.e. separation of the laminae, rotation of the bone, etc.

Treatment

In acute cases drugs are needed to reduce pain and make the animal more comfortable. Where the condition is suspected of being of digestive origin, bowel evacuation using mineral oils such as liquid paraffin is indicated.

More dramatic purgation with drugs such as dihydoxyanthraquinone is quick and effective in early cases and can bring a complete reversal of symptoms, especially in bigger horses. It is important to select cases for such treatment with care, but the removal of toxin-producing material from the gut is not only rational but essential.

Downward rotation of the third phalanx in laminitis. The gap that develops between sensitive and insensitive laminae (right) *is filled by blood and serum*

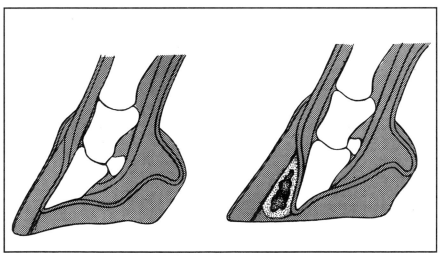

Other underlying causes, such as retained afterbirth, need intensive treatment as well as local treatment of the consequent laminitis.

Drugs of the NSAID type, of which phenylbutazone is the best known, are used for pain relief. Heparin and phenoxybenzamine have shown some effect in reversing the vascular changes within the foot. However, there is no universal agreement on the effectiveness of NSAID drugs and phenoxybenzamine itself is not licensed for use in the United Kingdom. Isoxuprine has also been used but its effect is unproven.

The condition has been treated with some success by physiotherapy in the form of pulsed electromagnetic fields, and because ultrasound and laser treatment also have remarkable effects on other conditions of the foot, these therapies may well prove to be a fruitful area in laminitis research.

Foot care is extremely important in restoring full use of affected animals to normal working life. This care may be helped by radiographs to establish horn growth and bone positioning. Corrective trimming is aimed at restoring the normal alignment of foot structures and limiting rotation of the pedal bone.

A heart-bar shoe helps this objective as do frog supports (these are available from proprietary sources, or can be made from cotton bandages and fitted under adhesive bandages).

Sand on the stable floor is found to reduce pain by providing a greater support for laminitic feet.

Prevention
When small ponies contract laminitis it is necessary to remove them from the source of their problem, grass. If lush grass growth is anticipated, susceptible animals should be kept on bare paddocks, or indoors, fed on hay only, then the condition is reasonably easy to avoid.

Laminitis in Thoroughbreds is uncommon where management is good, and, when it does occur, is normally satisfactorily reversed by relieving the symptoms and removing the cause. The use of a good purgative is a significant help in treating the Thoroughbred, especially where dietary elements are known to be the cause.

Osteochondritis Dissecans (OCD)

The term osteochondritis indicates inflammation of bone and cartilage. In OCD there is a tendency for pieces of cartilage to separate and enter the joint space.

Definition

This is a condition occurring in young horses in which abnormal development of cartilage and bone leads to synovitis and lameness. The disease develops through vascular defects causing erosion of cartilage and underlying bone. This causes joint inflammation with production of large amounts of synovial fluid. Affected joints are therefore usually enlarged.

Causes

Investigations into OCD in recent decades record a high incidence on individual farms and while it is suggested that there may be a hereditary element, this has not been proven.

The condition occurs most commonly in fast-developing Thoroughbred youngstock and there is an apparent relationship between incidence and nutrition. It has been identified in many joints although it is most common in the stifle and hock behind, and in the shoulder of the forelimb.

The disease has been diagnosed in foals, though this is unusual. The highest incidence is in two-year-old horses in training.

Signs

The common signs of OCD are joint enlargement and lameness, which may be intermittent. The condition is confirmed on radiography. More than one joint may be affected at the same time.

Weight increases the effect of concussion, therefore OCD of the shoulder is more common in males (on average the heavier sex) and heavier types of horses, suggesting an interplay between mechanical factors as well as development.

Treatment

Conventional therapies have little reported success with this condition, but cases treated by surgery have a good recovery rate. The damaged area is scraped clean using arthroscopy under general anaesthesia, and the joint flushed free of detrius. A significant number of animals return to full work after this procedure, following a recovery period of 6-12 months.

(Arthroscopic surgery is joint surgery using an arthroscope through which the joint can be observed. The technique allows for minimal interference with structures such as the joint capsule, and the surgery is carried out through very small incisions.)

Prevention

It is an important part of the management of young horses to be able to recognise when animals are growing too strongly, or when their development is unbalanced. Modern feed policies tend to press young horses to the limits of their growth potential, and very often to produce heavy-topped animals whose immature bones might not support this weight.

Prevention of OCD demands an understanding of nature's limits, and accepting a speed of growth that does not tax normal bone and cartilage formation.

Epiphysitis

The term epiphysitis (physitis) is recognised in common use relating to bone plate enlargements most commonly seen at the knee and fetlock. The epiphysis is the end of a lone bone, whereas the physis is the growth plate. On this basis, physitis is the more correct term, though the clinical condition seen has not changed.

Epiphysitis is described as abnormal development of a growth plate in a long bone. It is most noticeable in the lower growth plate of the radius just above the knee and in the lower growth plates of the metacarpus and metatarsus just above the fetlock.

Foal with epiphyseal enlargement at the lower end of the radius

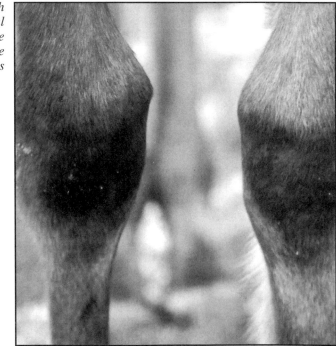

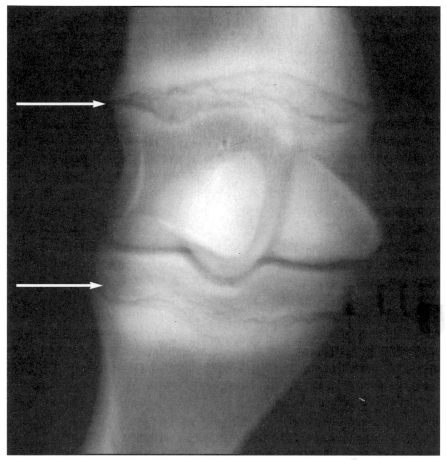

Radiograph showing epiphysitis in the fetlock joint of a foal

Causes
The condition is developmental in young foals but also occurs in any animal up to the stage of final bone maturation. It is commonly seen in strong, young growing foals, when it may be associated with rapid development combined with concussion at a time when body weight may be great in relation to bone strength. It is also common in big, backward two- and three-year-olds.

Signs
There is usually no lameness, but the enlarged growth plate is easily seen as a distortion of the part's normal anatomy. Movement may be restricted

and the animal may have a short, choppy action. This suggests low-grade pain rather than outright lameness. More than one leg is commonly affected.

The condition described as 'open knees' in two- and three-year-old horses is epiphysitis. In this case the lower radial growth plate is enlarged, creating the impression of abnormal space in the radiocarpal joint.

Treatment

It is important to check that the dietary intake of calcium, phosphorus and protein is balanced and to avoid over-feeding. The condition normally resolves itself with time if the animal is given a chance to develop without the added pressure of training or forced exercise.

Exertional Myopathies

Myopathy refers to disease of a muscle. In exertional myopathies the muscular problems arise with exercise and the severity of symptoms may directly relate to the effort.

This complex disease, with its variety of names (azoturia, tying up, setfast, etc.), was first recognised as 'Monday morning disease' because the condition was most common in working horses returned to work on Mondays. It has many grades today, indicating a number of underlying causes (hence the number of names), although all are marked by muscular involvement of some degree.

Causes

This is a disease of nutrition, circulation and the muscular system, caused by a number of factors some of which are already recognised and others which have not yet been established.

1) Typically, azoturia occurred in working horses which had been rested on Sundays while kept on full rations. The clinical condition which is still seen today is associated with high levels of lactic acid in the blood and marked pain and stiffness after a very short period in work.

2) A very similar condition occurs in the aftermath of some virus diseases. It is marked by hardening of the muscles, impaired gait and a failure to perform. On clinical grounds, there is good reason to believe this expression of the condition is preceded by liver disease.

3) The condition has also been associated with an inability to absorb minerals such as calcium, magnesium and sodium from the gut.

Signs

The animal may be short-striding on leaving its stable but may move normally. This may progress (or it can occur spontaneously) to a point where it stiffens and is unable to move. Profuse sweating and blowing occurs in acute azoturia. Muscles of the loins and quarters stiffen and become painful to touch. The urine may darken to a deep brown or bloody colour (due to the presence of myoglobin, a pigment found in muscles). There may be a rise in temperature.

In other conditions (tying up, setfast, etc.) the signs are similar to azoturia but variable in degree and intensity. Many horses are only mildly inhibited by the condition but are unable to be trained to racing standard. Riders complain that the horse is not extending properly, although lameness is slight. Abnormality in the muscles is always clinically evident in these cases and affected animals are frequently in poor condition.

Diagnosis is based on the symptoms and history of the animal. Blood tests taken at the time abnormality is apparent will show substantial rises in some serum enzyme levels - creatine kinase (CK) and aspartate aminotransferase (AAT) being examples.

Signs of muscle damage are visible on surface examination, and the animal has to be treated at once to relieve pain and other symptoms.

The reaction of muscle in this condition to electrical stimulation with a Faradic-type machine is typical when carried out after the acute symptoms have subsided; there is initial pain which soon passes off. This reaction is distinct from that in primary muscle injury in which muscle fibres are torn at exercise, when the injury to the muscle causes pain that responds to treatment over a period of time.

Treatment

In mild attacks the animal should be walked gently back to its stable or transport, but some horses cannot be moved except in a box or trailer.

Painkillers may be necessary to aid recovery and relieve the acute effects on afflicted muscle. Other drugs will neutralise symptoms, and judicious physiotherapy will help the animal to return to work within days.

The causes of this condition have become more complex with the passage of time and it is advisable to seek professional advice when it is recurrent.

Horses susceptible to azoturia should have their diet reduced when rested and should be warmed up gradually before hard work.

While electrical stimulation helps to disperse the accumulated waste products of exercise, it does not cure the condition. Complete cure depends on understanding the cause, eliminating it, and reversing the changes which have occurred in the blood.

The effects of lactic acid build-up in blood can be relieved clinically by administration of isotonic sodium bicarbonate solution intravenously. This frequently has a dramatic effect in acute azoturia and may allow animals to be returned to work without serious delay. When this works, the horse will often begin to move more freely as soon as the treatment has been completed. Many such horses can be ridden out the following day.

Horses which have suffered liver damage as a result of viral infections are often sensitive to large amounts of protein in their ration. Reduction of the level and quantity, or replacing high protein rations with oats, may have an added helpful effect.

Angular and Rotational Limb Deformities

Lameness is caused by a variety of deformities, some of which are discussed here.

Definition
A percentage of foals have limbs which deviate from normal at birth. This may occur on any limb and is most commonly exhibited as angulation of the carpus (knee), tarsus (hock) and fetlocks.

Limbs which deviate from normal: carpus valgus (left)*; carpus varus* (centre)*; a variation* (right) *of the same conditions*

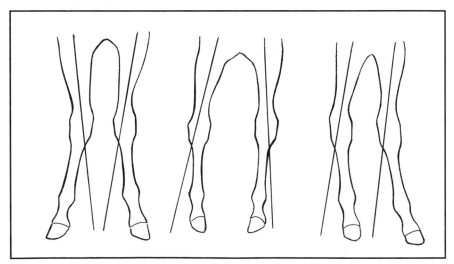

Depending on the direction of the angulation the condition is described in the following terms (using the carpus as an example): *carpus valgus* describes a situation where the knees are angulated inward and the limb from the metacarpus (cannon) down deviates outward; *carpus varus* is the opposite of this - the knee is directed outward and the lower limb inward. It is also not uncommon for the limb from the fetlock down to deviate inwardly in a *carpus valgus* situation, in which case the condition is described as *carpus valgus* and metacarpophalangeal (fetlock) joint *varus*. In this situation it is very likely that there will be some rotation of the large metacarpal (cannon) bone.

Causes
The condition is probably most common in premature foals when it is due to developmental weakness in the bone. It also occurs in mature, newly-born foals when it is suggested that it might result from positioning within the uterus.

The condition is also seen in growing foals when it arises owing to uneven development of the growth plates, possibly associated with poor foot angulation. This is distinct from epiphysitis (physitis), which generally occurs as a singular expression of development in older foals due to influences of weight and concussion on growing bone plates.

In some cases the development of this condition in foals of a few months old happens as a result of uneven weight bearing on developing bone at a time when the animal is growing vigorously. The initial problem may be precipitated by poor conformation of the feet which disturbs the natural limb axis and encourages abnormal growth.

The condition may also occur as a result of trauma, or as a consequence of lameness in a contralateral limb. Nutrition may also be a complicating factor.

Signs
The deformity of the limb is self-evident and may also involve some bone rotation, particularly of the metacarpus or metatarsus. Radiographs may be of help in identifying abnormal growth plate development.

Treatment
Affected foals are kept indoors as exercise is only likely to exacerbate the condition. Foot balance should be corrected by trimming as far as possible. Some cases respond to being placed in casts or braces if this is done in time, although care must be taken to avoid further injury (such as pressure ulcers) resulting from the cast.

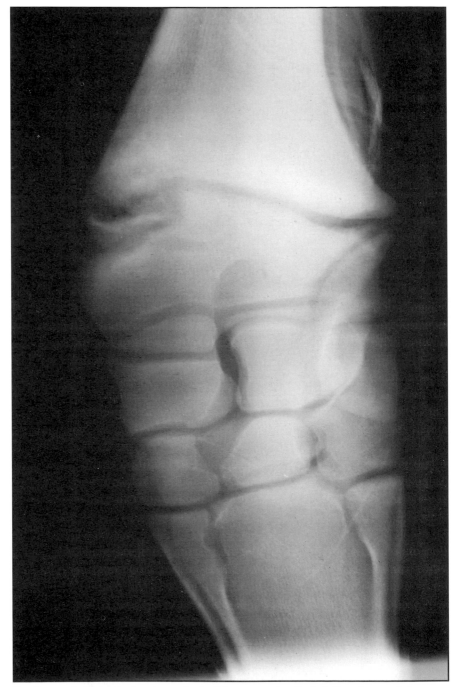

Radiograph (above) *showing a foal with an angular limb deformity; and the same limb* (opposite page) *with a staple inserted to correct the deviation*

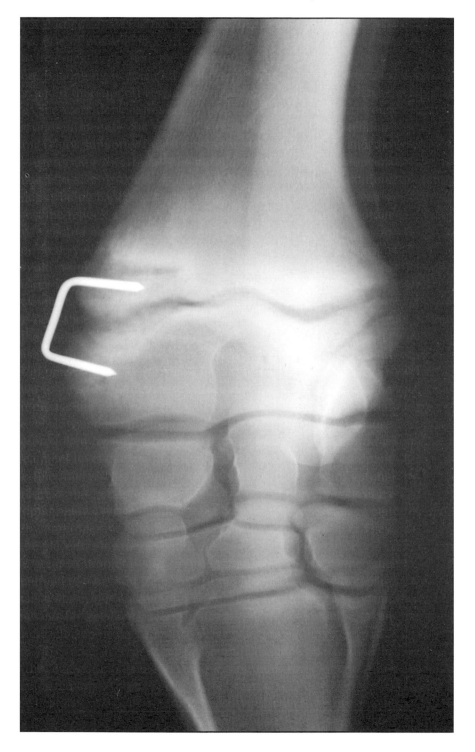

Surgery is necessary in cases that do not respond to conservative treatment. This is achieved by stripping the periosteum of the bone on the side away from the abnormal angulation in order to promote bone growth in that area and thus correct the imbalance (or problem). (In *carpus valgus* this would be done on the outer side of the lower end of the radius.) An alternative operation involves screwing or stapling the enlarged growth plate (the inner lower end of the radius on a *carpus valgus*) but the screws and staples must be removed when the deformity is corrected.

Prevention
This is only possible in more mature foals by detecting early signs of deformity and confining the animal immediately. Corrective trimming of the feet at an early stage may help prevent the condition from developing further.

Flexural Deformities

Previously linked with the term contracted tendons, flexural deformities are not uncommon in newborn or growing foals.

Definition
This condition occurs as a congenital condition in newborn foals and also as a developmental condition at a later stage. It may occur in a single limb

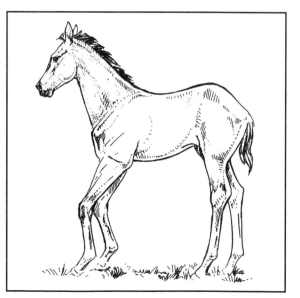

A foal with flexural deformity (contracted tendons). This type of deformity sometimes occurs in newborn foals and may correct itself without treatment

of the newborn but it is more likely to be bilateral in older foals. It may involve symptoms which relate primarily to the foot or, alternatively, to the fetlock.

Causes
In the newborn foal the condition is said to be due to foetal positioning within the mare and may resolve itself without treatment in a matter of days.

In older foals the condition is thought to occur owing to unbalanced relative growth of muscle (and tendon) and bone. Thus the bone may be long in relation to the length of the tendon and the effect is one of tendon contraction with varying degrees of deformity of the lower limb joints.

Signs
The condition is recognised by the angulation of the lower limb, and badly-affected foals may stand on their toes with boxy development of the feet. The pasterns are upright, the foot axis is broken forwards in many cases.

In older animals the fetlock joint may stand almost directly above the foot (without gross deformity of the foot itself). In extreme cases the knee (carpus) may be flexed.

It is important to establish that the presence of flexural deformities is not a secondary expression of some other problem, e.g. infection in the foot.

Treatment
In newborn foals flexural deformities may disappear in a matter of days; this process is often helped by allowing animals limited exercise to encourage use of their limbs.

Badly-affected foals may need assistance to suckle, and if confined to a large stable or barn may progress adequately without the problem of trying to keep abreast with their dams in an open field. Splinting the limb with padded guttering is often helpful in quickening the process.

Older foals are helped by corrective foot trimming, designed to lower the heels and restore foot balance. Surgery may be indicated in advanced cases, in which the inferior check ligament is sectioned. Fitting a shoe with a toe extension may prove helpful with an older animal. It is also important that the diet be checked and normal levels of minerals such as calcium and phosphorus be ensured.

Laxity of the flexor tendons also occurs as a common anatomical defect at birth. Affected foals frequently stand on their fetlocks with the

foot in exaggerated extension. The condition usually responds without treatment in a matter of days.

Nutritional Causes of Lameness

Lameness as a consequence of faulty nutrition occurs in a limited number of situations. It might be argued that a percentage of cases of OCD are primarily nutritional in origin, being due to excessive feeding inducing a rate of growth that places too great a strain on the bones. The lesions which develop are thus an expression of too great a body weight in comparison to bone strength.

Rickets is a long-recognised condition of bone which occasionally occurs in horses, and is due to faulty bone formation as a result of deficiencies or imbalances of calcium, phosphorus and vitamin D. External signs of rickets may not be easily identified because often there is no lameness and no deformity associated with it. Diagnosis may only be possible when a bone has shattered, or it may be picked up on radiography.

Nutritional secondary hyperparathyroidism (osteodystrophia fibrosa, or bran disease) occurs as a consequence of feeding excessive quantities of phosphorus. The result is abnormal bone development, and is often recognised clinically by abnormal instability of the knee when the animal is standing. Confirmation of the opinion is established when the diet is examined.

As stated earlier, malabsorption of calcium, magnesium and sodium from the bowel results in deficiencies within the body and is an implicated factor in some cases of exertional myopathy (azoturia). The diagnosis in this situation is clinically difficult and is assisted by blood and urine analysis. In some cases the mere correction of diet and supplementation of the deficient constituent may effect a cure. However, the cause may be more complicated and some cases do not respond.

Copper deficiency is considered important in some developmental conditions in young horses although there is not universal agreement on its influence. However, if copper deficiency is proven to exist in any developmental condition, supplementation is necessary by injection or orally.

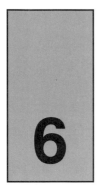

6 Lameness Related to Bursae, Sheaths, Tendons and Ligaments

The incidence of lameness is high in those structures of the horse we know as the bursae, sheaths, tendons and ligaments.

It should always be remembered, however, that, aside from direct trauma (such as a blow, or placing a foot in a hole) the occurrence of inflammation in such structures is often an expression of secondary lameness resulting from undetected abnormalities in other parts of the horse's anatomy.

Injury to Bursae and Sheaths

Bursae and sheaths are anatomical structures designed to reduce friction between moving parts. They possess synovial lining membranes which secrete a fluid similar in nature to joint fluid. Where a tendon, ligament or muscle passes over a bone, a bursa is interposed as a buffer to prevent damage to either structure.

Injury usually occurs as a result of trauma. This is marked by swelling of the bursa and often pain on manipulation. There may or may not be lameness.

True bursae exist in the shoulder (bicipital bursa) and over the great trochanter of the femur (trochanteric bursa). False bursae may develop wherever there is repeated irritation, on the hock, elbow or knee and are described as hygroma (because of fluid accumulation) of the elbow or knee, for example.

Bursitis may occur in other situations and is particularly common on the back, where ligament or muscle overlies bony prominences.

Sheaths are found around tendons, which they protect from wear and friction by benefit of their fluid secretion.

Capped Hock and Capped Elbow

These conditions, though different anatomically, are paired here because of their similar nature and cause.

Definition
These are bursal enlargements occurring at the point of the hock and the point of the elbow.

Causes
The condition is caused by repeated aggravation or trauma resulting in the development of a bursa. Capped hock usually results from striking the hock against a wall or partition and is frequently seen in horses that are bad travellers. Capped elbow is likely to arise from injury caused when the inner branch of the shoe strikes the elbow as an animal is lying down.

Signs
The swellings are characteristic, soft to the touch and painful and hot when they first appear. There is usually lameness only in the early stages, or if the bursa manages to become infected.

The right hock is capped

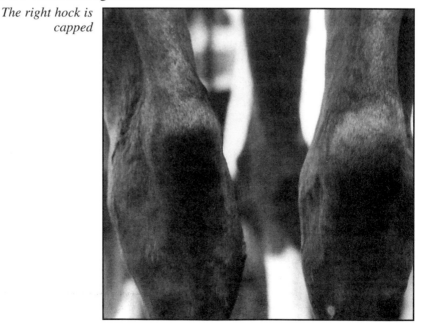

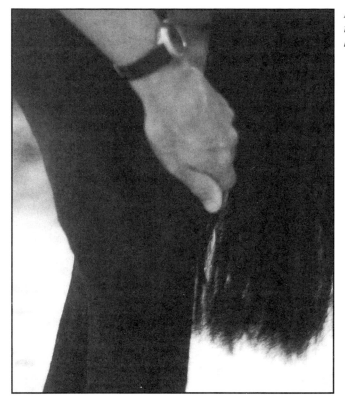

Detecting heat at the point of the hock

Treatment

Treatment is only necessary if the condition is chronic and causing lameness or if there is infection.

Non-infected bursae may be treated by draining and injection with an anti-inflammatory drug. (There are certain risks involved in using corticosteroids for horses and these must be taken into account.) Bursitis also responds well to drainage followed by laser or ultrasonic therapy (as long as there is no infection present).

Infected bursae require drainage and irrigation. Antibiotic therapy may also be of use.

Poll Evil and Fistulous Withers

These are infectious conditions that occur within bursae situated between the *ligamentum nuchae* and the bone at the poll and withers respectively. The condition is not common today and this reduction in incidence may have resulted from the success of brucellosis eradication in the United Kingdom and Ireland. In theory, any organism could cause infection of

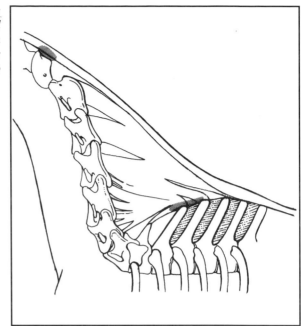

Position (shaded) *of the bursae at the poll and withers, in which poll-evil and fistulous withers develop*

these bursae, but vaccination against *Brucella abortus* (the causal organism) was effective in a high percentage of cases in the past; which also suggests that the organism gained entrance to the bursae through the blood.

Thoroughpin

Conditions that are expressed by soft tissue swellings in the region of the hock are common. They are distinguished by the anatomical positions in which they occur.

Definition
This is an inflammation of the deep flexor tendon sheath near the point of the hock. It is not to be confused with bog spavin which involves the lining of the joint itself.

Causes
The condition results from strain or trauma to the sheath.

Signs
Thoroughpin appears as a swelling on the upper posterior aspect of the

hock. The swelling occurs at a point which is higher than that for bog spavin. It is also distinguished by the fact that pressure applied to the swelling on the outside of the tendon only results in enlargement on the inner side. It does not cause any swelling to appear at the front of the hock, which would indicate the presence of fluid in the joint itself.

Treatment
The swelling usually reduces in size gradually and, normally, treatment is only given to showing animals to remove the blemish. The fluid is drained and the area injected with an anti-inflammatory drug or treated with laser or ultrasonic therapy.

Similar inflammation may occur to any other tendon sheath (e.g. the flexor or extensor tendons of the fore and hind limbs), and treatment, when required, will follow the same lines as above.

Injuries to the flexor tendon sheath above the fetlock may or may not be associated with injury to the tendon itself and this distinction needs to be made. Treatment here may involve the use of phenylbutazone and local therapy with laser or ultrasound. The horse should only be returned to work when the inflammation has disappeared and the leg is cold, reintro-

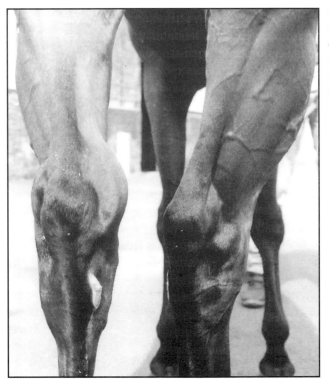

The swelling in thoroughpin occurs at the back of the limb, in front of the bony point of the hock (Photo: Sue Devereux)

ducing it to its work gradually and with great care. When in doubt about the basis of the condition ultrasound scanning can help to define its precise limits.

Windgalls

The term 'windgall' is long understood in equine literature relating to soft swellings in the fetlock region. Inevitably, science requires more specific terminology for the condition (idiopathic synovitis). However, the common name remains in everyday use.

Windgalls are found above the fetlock joint in all four limbs and may involve the tendon sheath (tendinous windgalls) or joint capsule (articular windgalls). Their presence indicates excessive synovial fluid accumulation in either structure.

When young animals are overused windgalls may occur, in which case they are a warning to exercise caution. In mature animals they are seen as blemishes only and have little clinical significance.

Causes
Windgalls in young horses are a result of a combination of immaturity, exercise and concussion. They persist in some horses throughout life and are seldom a source of lameness.

Signs
Articular windgalls are seen between the suspensory ligament and the back of the large metacarpal bone and represent a distension of the fetlock joint capsule.

Tendinous windgalls are identified between the back of the suspensory ligament and the deep flexor tendon at the upper limit of the fetlock.

Swelling of the affected structure with accompanying pain and lameness may occur in acute cases.

Treatment
These swellings are effectively treated when fresh with laser, ultrasound and various forms of electrotherapy. They reduce quickly and remain healed. Windgalls on older horses may not respond and are best left untreated when there is no heat and no lameness present,

The condition needs to be distinguished from more serious injury to the fetlock joint when presented in an individual limb, especially if there is lameness and heat on palpation. Radiographic examination will be required.

If young horses are working on hard ground, windgalls may develop quickly and be associated with heat and altered gait. This should be accepted for what it is: a warning of immaturity and impending bone/joint damage. The animal should be laid off work until the heat has disappeared and the joints have returned to normal.

Injuries to Tendons and Ligaments

Because of the dynamic nature of the horse and the special limitations of its leg anatomy, injury to tendons and ligaments has a particular importance. These types of problem occur in all kinds of ridden horses, but are most common in animals that race or jump competitively.

Tendons differ from ligaments in construction, attachments and function, but their place in the anatomy and physiology of the leg has much common ground. A tendon is not a separate entity, but an extension of the fleshy part of a muscle. It is strong and sinuous, and is attached into bone at its distal end. The fleshy part of the muscle is elastic and capable of contraction and relaxation; tendon has little elasticity and is almost rigid

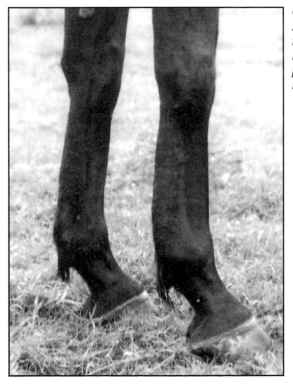

Chronic injury of the superficial flexor tendon of the right foreleg. Both limbs have been fired, a procedure now considered unprofessional

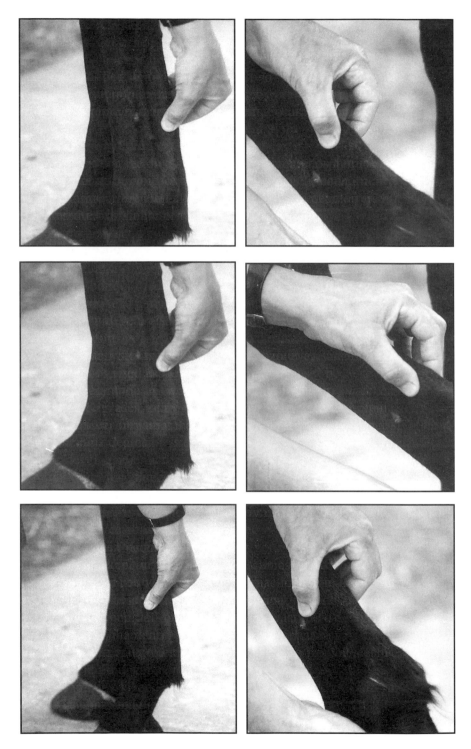

when compared with muscle. A tendon and its attached muscle act in unison to promote movement, bear weight and take stretch.

A ligament, on the other hand, originates from, and is attached to, bone. It is less flexible even than tendon.

Muscle fibre is more delicate and more capable of being strained than tendon. The difference in their respective healing properties, however, makes tendon injury a great deal more serious than muscle injury.

The most common site of tendon injury is to the flexors of the foreleg, in the area between the back of the knee and the fetlock. Different structures may be damaged here and the degree of injury varies from mild bruising to complete rupture of tendon fibres (even of an entire tendon body).

The most commonly injured ligament is the suspensory ligament, situated at the back of the metacarpal and metatarsal (cannon) bones, between the bone and the deep flexor tendon.

Anatomy

The tendons of the superficial and deep flexor muscles are outstanding features in the anatomy of the leg. The superficial tendon begins above the knee and is joined by a strong fibrous band, the radial or superior check ligament, which fuses with it at the back of the knee. It then continues down through the carpal canal in the carpal synovial sheath. In the cannon region it flattens and then widens into a ring above the fetlock through which the tendon of the deep flexor muscle passes. The superficial tendon divides into two parts below the fetlock, and attaches to either side of the hinder part of the first and second phalanges. The deep flexor tendon passes through this fork, within the digital synovial sheath, to be inserted into the third phalanx at the semilunar crest. The navicular bursa is interposed at this point, between the deep flexor and the distal sesamoid (navicular) bone.

The deep flexor tendon is formed above the knee and passes down through the carpal canal; it is united to the back of the knee by a 10cm fibrous band, the subcarpal or inferior check ligament which merges with the tendon about halfway down the cannon. When excessive strain falls

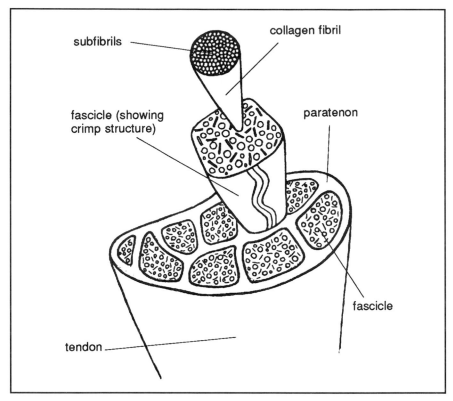

Tendon structure

on the deep flexor this ligament takes part of the weight and can be injured.

The two flexor tendons, one overlying the other, can be easily felt, but it is not always simple to separate them by touch.

Normal Tendon Structure

Tendons are composed of closely-packed bundles of collagen arranged parallel to one another but following a helical course along the length of the tendon. They produce a crimped (or wave) shape at the surface. Fibroblasts are arranged in long rows in the spaces between the collagen bundles but do not contribute to tendon strength. All collagen is replaced every six months.

The endotendon lies between the tendon bundles and carries the blood vessels, nerves and lymphatic vessels. It is an extension of the peritendon, outside which is the paratendon or the tendon sheath. The paratendon is elastic and pliable and allows the tendon to move backwards and forwards inside it.

Annular ligaments exist around the tendons at points where there is a risk that they might bend or bow-string.

Tendons have a a high tensile strength but restricted elasticity. The wave form of the collagen disappears at very low levels of extension (3 per cent) and rupture occurs at higher extensions (in the region of 8 per cent).

Tendon Repair

The rupture of the tendon collagen bundles is followed, as in any tissue destruction, by effusion of blood and serum into the gap created and a clot is formed. Reparation is made by invasion of the clot by fibroblasts and capillaries both from the peritendon and the endotendon. The manner in which new collagen bundles are laid down is random, not parallel as before, and exercise has a significant part to play in restoring the old design.

After injury, an acute inflammatory reaction lasts for about 48 hours followed by a phase lasting three to four weeks in which there is fibrous tissue deposition. The repair is then remodelled for the next three to four weeks. Repair thus reaches half strength in six to eight weeks but is not completed for a great deal longer than that.

This remodelling continues through the retraining period, which should not begin for six months, and it is critical that exercise is resumed slowly and built up steadily over a period of months. To restore tendon strength success is directly related to understanding and patience.

Causes of Tendon Injury
Injuries to tendons and the causes of same are numerous; some are itemised here.

1)   Excessive exercise when a horse is unfit, or incurred when trying to get it fit too quickly.

2)   Trauma, caused by hard, uneven or false ground (i.e. ground that is alternately hard and soft).

3)   Fatigue.

4)   When landing from drop fences.

5)   Slipping up.

6)   Bad conformation: long weak pasterns; back at the knee; tied-in below the knee.

7)   Muscular injury; this reduces the elasticity of the muscle/tendon unit and alters the flight of the leg.

8)   Over-reaches, too-tight bandages or boots, and other trauma.

Signs

A slight strain may affect the sheath and fibres of the superficial flexor tendon only, resulting in heat and a little swelling. There may be no lameness, but if the leg is picked up and the area subjected to light finger pressure, pain will be noted. It is important to distinguish between real pain and the resentment some horses show to any applied pressure. Where there is an injury the pain will be confined to the area in which there is heat. If in doubt, the reaction is compared with that of a sound leg.

A more severe strain with rupture of fibres will cause greater swelling, which may give the leg a bowed appearance and span most of the length of the tendon. Lameness is often present at the walk and pain is marked on finger pressure.

Rupture of a whole tendon will cause the fetlock to be dropped below its normal position. If both the superficial and deep tendons are ruptured, the fetlock will have lost the greater part of its support and may drop almost to the level of the ground. The horse will be in acute distress and the pain will cause it to sweat and blow.

The presence of heat in a tendon is a warning at any time that there is a weakness. Trainers feel the tendons and joints of their horses every evening to detect early signs of injury and horses found to have any heat are treated to special care. The more advanced injuries cannot easily be mistaken.

It is common today to examine injured tendons with diagnostic ultrasound scanners. This exercise is a useful adjunct to visual examination where there is doubt as to the extent of an injury or the state of repair.

Treatment

There are three phases in tendon repair: the immediate control of the inflammatory response; the period of rest; and the return to work.

Each phase is important and needs to be clearly understood if a return to full work is to be achieved.

1)   In any tendon injury it has to be appreciated that the mechanics of leg anatomy tend to draw the injured ends apart. For this reason support of the injury is vital in the early stages. Efforts to limit the inflammation vary, involving the use of heat (in the form of poultices), cold hosing or ice. In addition, NSAID drugs are used (e.g. phenylbutazone, which may be necessary to control reaction and pain in severe cases).

The use of corticosteroids is not recommended, either locally or systemically, because of possible side effects.

Whatever treatment is applied, the initial inflammatory response has to be controlled. Bandaging is essential to limit swelling for the first two to three weeks, and if this support is withdrawn too early the problem can be made worse. The work done at this stage decides the extent of the fibrous tissue repair and, ultimately, the size and strength of the repaired tendon. If the tendon is not supported, the reaction will be far greater and the chances of it returning to a relatively normal size are greatly reduced. Allowing nature to take its course is not a wise move with this condition.

When a leg is being bandaged, it is important to apply pressure evenly and to support the fetlock as well when the injury is near the joint. Cotton wool or gauze should be placed under non-adhesive support bandages to prevent interference with blood supply. When using adhesive bandages it is vital to avoid wrinkling or twisting of the bandage material. It is also wise to give support to both injured and sound legs in order to avoid damage to the weight-bearing leg.

A wedge-heel shoe may be applied for the first few weeks to relieve tension on the tendon. Some veterinarians advocate the use of plaster casts to immobilise the limb and prevent further damage. However, this should only be left in place for the initial phase of repair.

About two to three days after the initial injury, the injured area can be treated with ultrasound or laser therapy. It is important to keep the initial treatment levels low and to only treat the perimeters of the injury, because pain can be provoked by treatment at this stage. In another two to three days, the treatment level can be increased and the treatment head brought directly over the injury. This is one of the most effective ways of getting a good repair, the aim being to minimise swelling and prevent adhesions from developing. However, a warning must be given: severe damage can be caused by improper or injudicious use of these instruments. They should not be placed in inexperienced hands.

2)   The greatest problem with slight tendon injuries arises when the animal is returned to work too soon, before the leg has had time to repair. Some animals with serious tendon injuries continue to race effectively, but they are few and far between. Every injury to this area should be taken seriously and each step of the return to work watched with care.

After the first three or four weeks, the animal should be walked in hand, with the leg well bandaged, once or twice daily for about 30 minutes. This helps the repair process.

When the heat has gone and the animal is sound it should be turned out and given a period of not less than six months rest before being returned to work. The healing of tendon tisuue takes a considerable time to complete.

Tendon injuries are very often preceded by muscular damage, and if this has happened it is critical that the muscle be treated before the horse is put back into work, otherwise the condition is almost certain to recur.

Excellent results with injured tendons are achieved through intelligent use of physiotherapy.

The cause of the initial injury has to be established and, where possible, recurrence avoided. But the majority of horses will continue to work sound if the mechanics of the condition, and the animal, are fully taken into account.

3)   While a variety of mild (and strong) blisters are used when the horse is not working, their effect is questionable. Time, and judicious exercise, will restore the tendon to a state which is close to its former strength. The return to work must be slow and patient, with weeks of walking before an animal trots, and weeks of trotting before it canters. Ideally the introduction to faster gaits should take three to six months, and patience is well rewarded.

It is important to appreciate the changes that occur in body structures during training, before a state of fitness is reached. After injury, there is continuing reorganisation within injured tissues as repair is being completed. Thus strength is restored and the tendon continues to reduce in size from its post-injury swollen condition. A high percentage of horses treated with understanding remain sound. Those that are not given this chance may well break down again.

Most surgical (principally tendon-splitting and carbon-fibre implants) and injection techniques have failed to prove statistically that they are any better than conservative forms of treatment for injured tendons. Furthermore, any procedure that increases reaction and which leaves an animal with an unavoidable swelling is less likely to provide the strength to withstand training than one that does not.

There is a great deal of controversy over the treatment of tendon injuries, especially when the condition is chronic. The Royal College of Veterinary Surgeons (RCVS) has banned the firing of horses, and this action deserves support.

A number of drugs have been used for local treatment of tendon injuries. Among these are hyaluronic acid and polysulfated glycosamino-glycans (PSGAG), both of which have shown useful properties in the treatment of joint conditions. Their effectiveness in tendon injuries remains unproven and does not appear to provide any benefits over conservative treatment, although recent claims for PSGAGs used intramuscularly have yet to be evaluated.

Di-methyl sulfoxide (DMSO) has shown itself capable of reducing the local inflammatory response (used superficially) in the early days after injury and in encouraging reduction of swelling. Methyl-sulphonyl methane (MSM) is a natural derivative of DMSO and has a similar effect when given orally.

Where one or both flexor tendons have been severed fully, surgery is sometimes performed to join the parted ends together. In this situation there may be some benefit to be had from carbon-fibre implants to help support the damaged structures. However, such animals are saved for breeding purposes through conventional treatment, by providing adequate support to both injured and weight-bearing limbs, by controlling pain and allowing an extended period for recovery. Some animals are humanely destroyed because of their suffering.

Superficial Flexor Tendon Displacement (Hock)

In this condition the injury that occurs is not within the tendon itself but to the support structures that hold it in position in an anatomically vulnerable area.

Definition
The superficial flexor tendon passes over the point of the hock, to which it is attached by fibrous bands. Damage to either of these bands allows the tendon to become displaced to either side, though usually medially. The condition is most common in racehorses.

Causes
It may be linked with poor conformation and occurs most commonly as a result of trauma during the course of a jumping race or when galloping.

Signs
There is marked lameness and swelling occurs at the point of the hock after a matter of hours. Initially the injury may be identified from the abnormal positioning of the tendon on the hock.

Once swelling has developed, the condition may not easily be distinguished from capped hock, though, as it reduces, the abnormal placing of the superficial flexor tendon is seen. It must not be confused with rupture of the Achilles tendon at the point of the hock or damage to other structures of the joint.

Treatment

Many horses recover with extended rest, though there is a risk that the condition may recur and the animal's action may be permanently influenced by it. This makes the likelihood of further complications more probable.

Surgery is sometimes carried out, and with varying degrees of success.

Injury of the Suspensory Ligament (Desmitis)

Desmitis is injury of any ligament. As we have already seen, the difference between tendon and ligament is that ligament has no muscular attachment and only connects bone to bone. However, the suspensory ligament differs from other ligaments in its basic construction.

Between the deep flexor tendon and the cannon (large metacarpal) bone the suspensory ligament is a flat, elastic band about 25mm wide which takes origin from the back of the knee, then passes down the limb, occupying the channel between the back of the cannon bone and the splint

The division of the suspensory ligament and attachment to the sesamoid bones. The arrows indicate the most common sites of injury

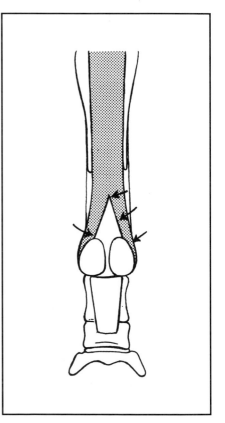

(small metacarpal) bones. Like all structures behind the cannon it is subject to strain.

At the level of the sesamoid bones it divides and sends two branches forward to join the extensor tendon on the front of the pastern. The rest of the ligament is attached to the sesamoid bones themselves. The function of the suspensory ligament is to suspend the fetlock and support the leg, although it is also concerned with preventing dorsiflexion (over-extension) of the fetlock joint.

The suspensory ligament is part of the stay apparatus. It is unusual in that it is a modified muscle, containing some muscle tissue and possessing considerable elasticity when compared with other ligaments. In supporting the joint it is aided by the tendons of both superficial and deep flexor muscles. Together with the proximal sesamoid bones it carries most of the weight of the horse at many stages of locomotion.

Definition
Injury to the suspensory ligament occurs as a primary injury, usually where the branches attach to the sesamoid bones or at the point of division in the lower third of the metacarpal area. Injury to this ligament differs from that to the flexor tendons because of:
1)   A different anatomical structure.
2)   Different mechanical functions in the limb.
3)   Differences in repair of the tissues involved.

Causes
Injury is probably due to over-extension of the fetlock joint, causing over-stretching of the suspensory ligament. Hard or uneven ground are causal factors, as is fatigue, because in this state the fetlock tends to drop closer to the ground at fast gaits.

Signs
There is diffuse swelling of the full tendon area, and pain on palpation of the ligament itself. The horse will be lame and have a short choppy stride at the trot. Heat and swelling may be marked, and the condition is best identified with the leg picked up so it can be distinguished from injury to other structures. There is no bowing of the outer tendons and no pain when the flexors are subjected to finger pressure. An injured suspensory usually has a soft feeling to it when compared with the ligament of a sound leg.

It is important not to confuse tendon and ligament injuries with infection of the same area, which can be equally painful and cause similar types

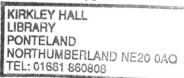

of swelling. Radiographs should be taken where there is a possibility of damage to the sesamoid bones. Ultrasonic scanning can help to distinguish suspensory ligament and tendon injuries.

Treatment
Support by bandaging is important initially, together with other measures to limit pain and control the extent of the inflammatory process. After the first two days the ligament may be treated with ultrasound or laser therapy and, in uncomplicated cases, the horse will gradually be introduced to walking exercises after a few weeks. Many return to full work in six weeks to three months.

Repair of the suspensory ligament is very different from that of the flexor tendons because of the dynamic influences of limb anatomy and the nature of the tissues involved. The principles of repair in any lower limb injury mean that support of the limb should aim to hold the injured parts together. While this is not easily achieved in tendon repair (because of the nature of tendon construction) it is a basic principle in any situation involving ligaments.

The purpose of physiotherapy, then, is to stimulate natural healing and to return the part to full use through judicious exercise when the repair has achieved adequate strength.

Sprain of the Carpal Check Ligament

The term 'check ligament' describes a fundamental purpose of this structure to limit movement of the tendon to which it is attached. It varies from other ligaments in that it connects bone to tendon.

This is a short ligament that extends from the back of the knee to the deep flexor tendon, about halfway down the cannon bone. It supports the deep tendon and also plays a part in the stay apparatus. There is also a radial check ligament which is part of the same apparatus; however, it is less commonly involved in lameness.

Causes
The most likely cause of injury is sudden over-extension of the knee.

Signs
Lameness is not very marked, the horse tends to prop slightly and shorten its stride on the affected leg.

Heat and swelling are detected at the back of the knee and there is pain on manipulation of the injured ligament.

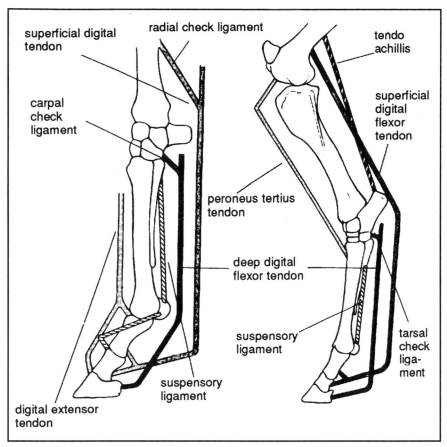

superficial digital
tendon

radial check ligament

tendo
achillis

carpal
check
ligament

superficial
digital
flexor
tendon

peroneus tertius
tendon

deep digital
flexor tendon

suspensory
ligament

tarsal
check
liga-
ment

suspensory
ligament

digital extensor
tendon

The carpal check ligament, in relation to the tendons of the foreleg (left) *and the tendons of the hind leg* (right)

Treatment

The condition responds well to either ultrasound or laser therapy as long as the horse is rested. The animal should not be ridden until all heat has gone from the area because the structures at the back of the knee are under constant strain and full repair is essential.

It is difficult to support this ligament, so rest and judicious exercise are imperative.

Curb (Sprain of the Plantar Ligament of the Hock)

Like windgall, 'curb' is a term in common use. While its meaning is specifically defined, a full understanding of the nature of the condition requires knowledge of the anatomy involved.

Curb (right) *occurs on the line from the point of the hock to the fetlock* (Photo: Sue Devereux)

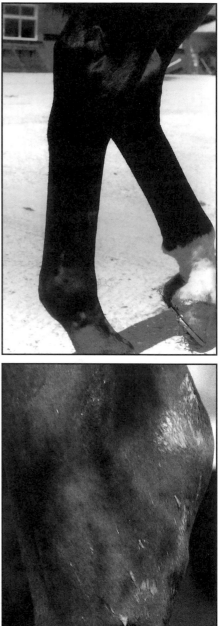

An overbent hock (below, left) *with a tendency to curb formation; swelling at the back of the hock* (below, right) *is higher here than is normal for a curb. However, it would still be referred to as a curb*

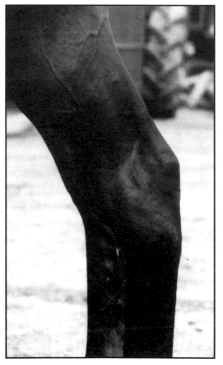

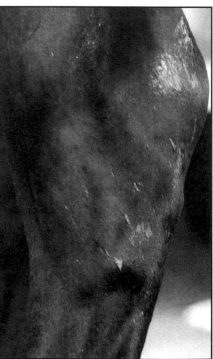

This is a strain of the ligament binding the hock (tarsus) to the cannon bone at the back of the hind limb. It is defined as any deviation in a straight line from the point of the hock to the fetlock situated at the lower end of the hock (although this is not wholly correct).

Strain of the ligament is frequently followed by bony enlargement at the lower end of the hock which makes the blemish permanent.

Causes
The condition is a result of over-flexion of the hock joint when in a weight-bearing position.

Horses with badly made, weak hocks are predisposed to the condition. It is also caused by working and/or jumping under-developed immature horses unfit for the work.

Curb is also a recurring problem in trotters and pacers.

Signs
The swelling is best seen with the horse's leg viewed from the side. If the head of the splint bone is enlarged or positioned slightly behind the perpendicular line, this does not constitute a curb (this is sometimes called 'false curb', a term which is also used to describe a bursal enlargement at the same site).

Lameness may be noted in the early stages but it is short-lived and mild in character. The typical swelling will be found on the midline at the lower end of the back of the hock. There will be heat and pain initially but this soon passes. The enlargement may become bony and continue to grow if the hock is weak and under continuous strain.

Treatment
Many curbs require no treatment, although the swelling is considered to be a serious blemish for showing purposes and owners will request treatment for this reason. Early swelling is best treated with ultrasound or laser, and the hock should not be subjected to any sudden strains until all heat has gone from the site. Larger swellings with poorly-made hocks and bony invasion of the curb are unlikely to be improved by any form of treatment. As long as the animal is sound the problem is best ignored.

Sprain of the Distal Sesamoidean Ligaments

The sesamoidean ligaments are typical ligaments that connect bone to bone. They form part of the stay apparatus; there are nine sesamoidean ligaments including the suspensory ligament.

The position (blacked in) *of the distal sesamoidean ligament*

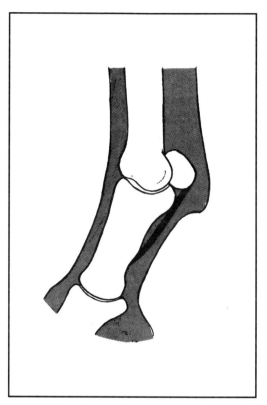

Definition
The distal sesamoidean ligaments connect the lower surface of the sesamoids to the back of the first phalanx. Injury may cause swelling at the back of the pastern and lameness.

Causes
Over-extension of the fetlock is the most likely cause, or any form of direct trauma.

Signs
Heat, swelling, and pain may be detected in the region at the back of the pastern, although swelling is naturally limited by the strong overlying tissues in this area. Radiographs may be used to confirm the diagnosis and to eliminate bony injury in the region.

Treatment
Ultrasound and laser therapy are useful with this type of injury if the region is well supported and the animal rested until repair is complete.

Deposition of bone during repair, however, may inhibit movement and influence future soundness.

Constriction of the Annular Ligament of the Fetlock

Essential structures that bear great burdens in locomotion, like the fetlock, knee and hock, are strengthened by annular ligaments.

Definition
The annular ligament of the fetlock surrounds the joint and encloses the superficial and deep flexor tendons; the superficial flexor also forms a ring here through which the deep flexor descends to the foot. Constriction of the annular ligament causes a characteristic deformation of the contour of the tendon above the fetlock and it inhibits natural movement.

Causes
Trauma to the fetlock itself is the most likely cause of this condition.

The surface deformity here encompasses the annular ligament area and partial loss of joint support suggests the ligament was ruptured at an earlier time

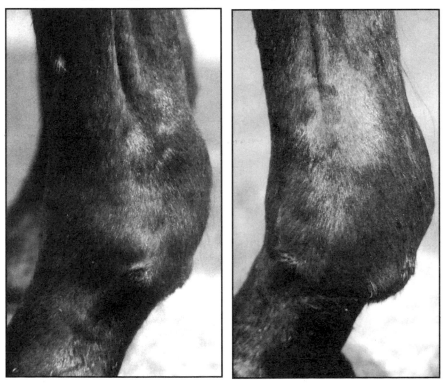

Signs

Constriction often becomes evident as a secondary problem after a substantial strain of the joint, or when the tendons under the annular ligament have repaired.

There may or may not be adhesions associated with it involving other structures (such as the tendons).

Treatment

Conservative treatment is unlikely to have any significanct effect on the condition once established. Surgery offers some hope in a percentage of cases.

The condition might be avoided by more effective treatment of the initial injury.

Carpal Tunnel Syndrome

A syndrome is where a number of clinical signs result from one cause. It is, too, a term used to describe a situation where the horse's symptoms are not specific and accurate diagnosis is elusive (e.g. the poor performance

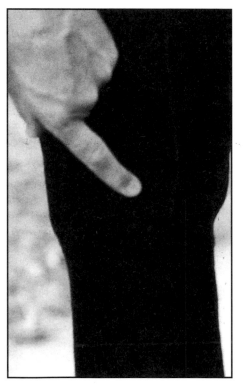

Indicating the area of the carpal tunnel

syndrome; but horses lose form for a variety of reasons and use of the term here is questionable).

At the back of the knee, the superficial and deep flexor tendons pass through the carpal tunnel, formed by the joint capsule in front and the annular ligament behind. Inflammation of the canal can cause constriction of the ligamentous structures over the tendons.

Causes
The condition is caused by trauma of the knee structures, with chronic tightening of the carpal tunnel.

Signs
There is constriction over the tendons at the back of the horse's knee with possible synovitis of the carpal sheath surrounding the tendons.

Carpal tunnel syndrome may cause a minor partial flexion of the knee and heat will be evident over the area in the early stages. Protraction of the limb is likely to be affected with shortening of the stride in its anterior phase.

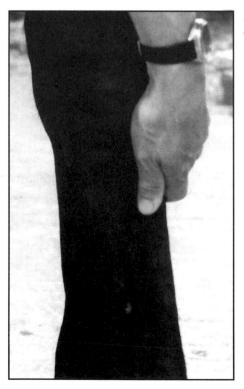

Feeling for heat in the carpal tunnel area

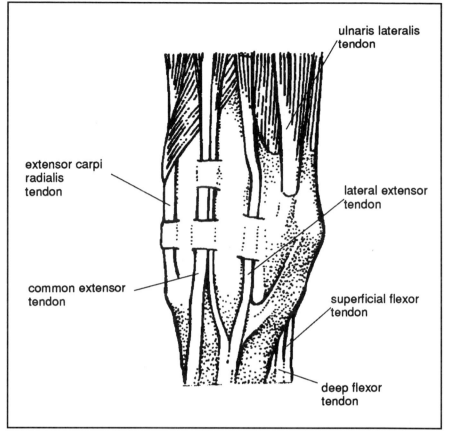

At the back of the carpus, the flexor tendons pass through the carpal tunnel formed by the joint capsule in front and the annular ligament behind

Treatment

Although carpal tunnel syndrome is not common in horses, it is unlikely to be successfully treated without surgery to relieve the constriction on the tendons.

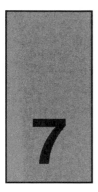

7 Lameness Associated with Joints

Lameness associated with joints is extremely common. This occurs for a variety of pathological reasons.

Joint Anatomy

The anatomical design of all limb joints is similar; differences being mainly a result of the type of movement required. The end of each long bone is dense to withstand the effects of concussion absorbed by a joint. The articular surfaces of these bones (the ends that meet their neighbours

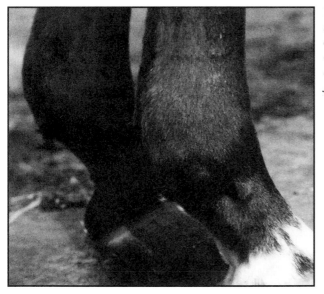

The fetlock joint here has lost detail due to bony enlargements which signify developing joint disease

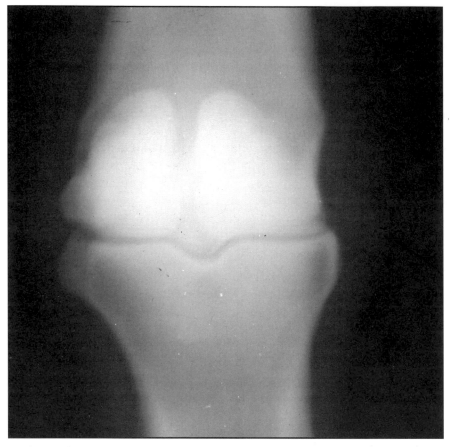

Radiograph of a fetlock joint; the horse has chronic joint trouble. The joint cavity is diminished, indicating developing joint disease

within a joint) are covered by a layer of cartilage, a substance of greater elasticity than bone. Its purpose is to protect the bone and reduce the chances of fracture occurring. Cartilage is without nerve supply and it obtains its nutrients through the synovial fluid of the joint. For this reason cartilage has limited ability to repair and any impairment of its nutrition (through changes in synovial fluid) will result in degeneration.

Synovial fluid, produced by the synovial membrane lining the joint capsule, is similar in constitution to blood plasma but with the significant addition of hyaluronic acid.

Hyaluronic acid, because of its large molecular size, is responsible for the viscosity of the fluid and its removal changes the fluid from a normal egg-white consistency to that of water. The purpose of synovial fluid is to lubricate the joint and nourish the cartilage.

As both the synovial membrane and the joint capsule have direct nerve and blood supplies, injury to either structure results in pain, either through direct tissue damage or from distension due to excessive production of synovial fluid.

This pain is expressed by lameness and resentment of passive movement; it is usually associated with heat and swelling which is detectable externally.

The joint capsule is attached to the periosteum of the bones making up the joint, so that in injury these attachments may be disrupted. The joint itself is further supported by collateral ligaments, or (as in the shoulder) muscle bodies. When the capsule and ligaments are injured this further complicates joint injury because the repair process may give rise to bony enlargements that subsequently affect joint movement.

The first principles, therefore, in confronting joint injuries are:
1)   Full diagnosis (including radiography, where required).
2)   Immobilisation of the part, where this is possible, and fostering union between separated tissues.
3)   Stimulation of natural repair processes. To neglect any of these is to invite chronic joint changes.

Primary Joint Trauma (Sprain)

The normal functioning of any joint depends on anatomical integrity. After injury, this normally will not be restored if the consequences of the repair process interfere with movement.

Definition
Primary joint trauma is injury to a joint and/or its related structures (capsule and collateral ligaments), due to external factors.

Causes
The circumstances under which sprains and strains to individual joints occur are as follows:
1)   Fast-pace work on uneven ground, or placing a limb in a hole.
2)   As a result of poor conformation or bad shoeing.
3)   Sudden corrective movements, as when an animal is pushed sideways at speed by another horse.
4)   Bad ground conditions when landing from a fence.
5)   Trotting persistently on a camber, or as the result of unevenly-wearing shoes.

Signs
There is usually heat and swelling of the affected joint, with marked lameness and pain on passive movement (moving the affected area by hand, with the limb off the ground).

Where there is any doubt as to the extent of the injury or the structures involved, radiography is essential. In many cases, the degree of initial pain and impressions of damage estimated on surface examination will dictate this.

Injury to the collateral ligaments may lead to joint instability and create the risk of luxation (dislocation), if the joint is not fully immobilised.

Treatment
The first principles of treatment are support for the joint, pain relief (when required), rest, and stimulation of the normal healing processes with ultrasound, laser or other forms of physical therapy. The application of cold (by ice or waterboot) may be effective in relieving the immediate inflammation. As a general rule, the body is capable of repairing any injured tissues if these are held in apposition and movement of the part is restricted in the early days after injury.

While the degree of damage will influence a decision, some injuries benefit from early limited exercise and others do not. Pain can be an excellent guide in deciding on this and any animal that improves with restricted walking is unlikely to be harmed by it. Those that do not may require more detailed investigation and should not have exercise imposed on them until the full extent of the injury is appreciated.

The use of NSAID drugs can be decided on the basis of symptoms and the need for pain relief. However, it should be appreciated that the suppression of pain often allows unwarranted use of injured parts and can result in more serious injury.

Degenerative Joint Disease (DJD)

The terms used to describe this osteoarthritic condition signify adverse changes in joint cartilage, in the bone (especially at the joint margins), and also in the synovial membrane.

Definition
In this condition degeneration of cartilage may follow changes in the synovial fluid due to inflammation of the synovial membrane and/or the joint capsule. This may be further aggravated by breakdown products of carti-

lage degeneration (proteoglycans) adding to the pathological process already established. Bony changes occur subsequent to cartilage degeneration.

Causes
The most probable initiating factor is direct trauma to the joint. However, this kind of joint disease may also ensue from conformational defects in the formation of a joint or as a result of excessive direct concussion.

DJD is more often seen as an expression of joint disease in older horses although it may occur in young horses, particularly those which are involved in racing. It is a condition that is generally progressive and irreversible, especially when established. It is commonly seen in the knee of racehorses, because of the particular forces this structure comes under during fast-pace work. The joints from the knee and hock downwards are more commonly affected than those above, again indicating that the cause is at least partly concussive.

Signs
There is usually enlargement of the joint capsule due to increased synovial production. Chronic changes to the anatomical structures involved may restrict movement and will usually increase lameness when the joint is flexed.

Externally the joint may show capsular or bony enlargement and heat is detected when the condition is aggravated. (Heat may not be detected in animals which have been rested for a period, but symptonms of lameness will return with exercise or following a period of rest after exercise.)

When examining any horse with recognisable joint deformity it is vital to subject that joint to adequate testing to judge its soundness. Radiographs may also be required in order to form an opinion. In the early stages of disease, however, no changes may show on a radiograph, but there may be heat and swelling on palpation and pain might well be detectable on passive movement of the joint. In other cases there are no signs except for lameness, and the joint flexes normally.

Radiographic changes include narrowing of the joint space due to cartilage destruction, degeneration of underlying bone and the production of bone growths on the edges of the articular surface.

Treatment
The first principle of any treatment is to remove evident underlying causes such as anatomical deformities; these might be helped by corrective shoeing. It is also important that joint injuries receive quick and correct

treatment so that the chances of chronic problems developing are minimised. The use of therapeutic ultrasound, laser and electromagnetic-field therapy at an early stage often effects a total cure as long as an animal is not returned to work before the healing process has been completed. The biggest risk with these procedures is that the reduction of inflammation and removal of pain may make it appear that the condition is healed before it actually is. It is vital, therefore, as long as there is any residual heat in the joint that the animal receive only controlled exercise and be confined to its box.

In chronic joint disease the condition may well be irreversible although various forms of therapy may reduce the inflammation, relieve pain and so allow an animal to be used.

First, the various forms of physical therapy, by relieving pain, allow an animal to continue an active life without, perhaps, having a great deal of influence on the underlying pathology.

Second, NSAID drugs may allow similar use without influencing the clinical condition either. While phenylbutazone is used with considerable safety in horses of conventional size, it can produce unacceptable side effects in ponies treated for prolonged periods. Therefore, there are vital considerations when any long-term medication is planned.

In addition, it must not be forgotten that the use of painkilling drugs may allow further destruction of already damaged tissues and that there is a risk of injuries to remote parts in a proportion of cases. Furthermore, the painkilling effect is not total and their success in this disease depends on the degree of injury.

When injected into injured joints sodium hyaluronate and PSGAG have a reparative effect; also when injected parenterally by a vet. Their purpose is to bring back normality to the synovial fluid and through this promote repair of damaged cartilage and restore normal joint function. Their use may be decided on the basis of synovial fluid analysis as well as on the persistence of symptoms. However, while these drugs are an effective method of treatment for DJD, their use is limited by expense. Neither are they cure-alls and in some situations their influence is short-lived.

Infectious Arthritis (Joint-ill in Foals)

Joints are normally sterile, but, because of the nature of synovial fluid, they offer a rich medium for the growth of organisms.

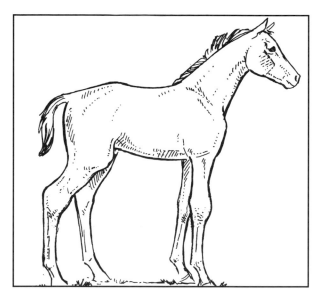

In joint-ill, it is not uncommon for swellings to develop in more than one joint. The fetlock, stifle, hock and knee joints are most commonly affected. Infection may also exist in pastern, elbow, shoulder and hip joints

Definition

Infectious arthritis occurs in adult animals most commonly as a result of penetrating wounds. In foals, the condition occurs in the immediate post-natal period by blood-borne infection contracted at birth and is often a consequence of poor immunity due to inadequate, or failed, colostrum transfer from the mare.

Signs

In the adult, infection is associated with acute lameness, pain, swelling, and often a raised temperature. In severe cases the animal may suffer loss of appetite.

Joint-ill, in so much as joint signs are the extension of a systemic infection, may well be preceded by loss of appetite, temperature, lassitude, and refusal to suck. When joint swelling is evident the condition may well be advanced.

The infection damages the synovial membrane, cartilage and bone. Diagnosis may be made on the basis of the symptoms and on the nature of the synovia (which may well leak from an open wound on an affected joint).

Infected synovia is discoloured and may be purulent or produce an offensive smell. The history of the case will also suggest a diagnosis and blood analysis will reveal high white blood cell counts and high fibrinogen levels.

Foal joints may rupture and pour infected material to the outside.

Alternatively, the synovial fluid may be drawn off and examined micro-scopically if there is any doubt. Infected fluid will be identified by the number and type of white blood cells contained in it and organisms may be seen under a microscope. However, it may not be easy to culture an offending organism from this source, but a negative result does not mean there is no underlying infection.

Treatment
Intensive antibiotic treatment is necessary to combat joint infections in adult animals. This may have to be started even before the organism can be identified and a sensitivity test carried out, by use of broad-spectrum cover.

It may also be necessary to flush the joint regularly to remove infected material and joint detritus.

In the case of a foal suffering from joint-ill, the first important factor is the supplementation of immunity by transfer of plasma from the dam. This quite simple procedure can be carried out without complicated equip-ment. Intensive antibiotic therapy is also necessary to overcome the infec-tion. While some foals make a complete recovery, many do not. In some cases, humane destruction is necessary to prevent suffering.

Individual Joints

The joints of the limbs and spinal column are sometimes classified by movement.

An arthroidal joint is one in which the bone surfaces are practically flat and in which there is only limited movement (e.g. the carpometacarpal joint between the lower row of knee bones and the cannon).

A ginglymus joint is a hinge joint in which movement is typically flex-ion and extension. Such a joint is the elbow, or the tibiotarsal joint (the upper joint of the hock).

A trochoid joint is one in which one bone rotates around another (e.g. the atlantoaxial joint in the neck).

An enarthrosis is a ball-and-socket joint (e.g. the hip). This type of joint has the greatest range of movement, but the extent of movement in the hip joint in the horse is limited by ligaments.

A diarthroidal joint (also called a synovial joint) is any joint in which there are two articular surfaces, a synovial membrane and a joint capsule. It is a general term that includes most joints in the body, including the above-mentioned joints.

Forelimb

In describing detail of the forelimb joints we will start at the foot and work upwards.

Coffin Joint

Type: Ginglymus.
Movement: Flexion and extension. Limited rotation on manual movement.
Bones: Second and third phalanges and distal sesamoid bone.
Anatomical structures: Joint capsule, two collateral ligaments, two collateral and one distal ligament of distal sesamoid.

Conditions
1)   Strain of the joint or related anatomical attachments.
2)   DJD, including low ringbone.

Conditions of neighbouring structures (for differential diagnosis)
1)   Infection of the foot, which may involve bone or structures such as the navicular bursa.
2)   Navicular disease.
3)   Pedal osteitis.

Detail of the coffin joint showing relationships within the foot and the position of the important ligaments

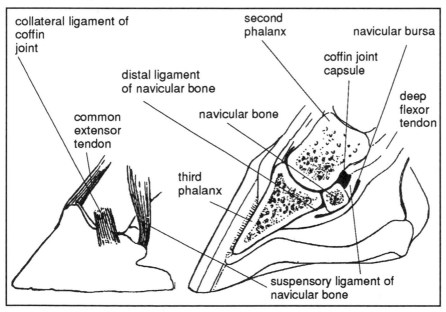

4) Laminitis.
5) Buttress foot and pyramidal disease.
6) Sidebone.
7) Trauma of sensitive sole, including corns.
8) Fracture of pedal and navicular bones.
9) Keratoma.

Pastern Joint

Type: Ginglymus
Movement: Limited flexion and extension with a minor degree of rotation possible on passive movement.
Bones: First and second phalanges.
Anatomical structures: Joint capsule, two collateral ligaments and four palmar ligaments.

Conditions
1) Strain of joint or related attachments.
2) DJD (including high ringbone)

The pastern joint (left) *and its ligaments* (right)

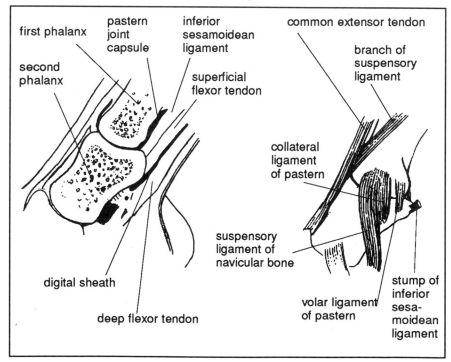

Conditions of neighbouring structures
1)   Strain of inferior sesamoidean ligaments.
2)   Fractures of first and second phalanges.

Fetlock Joint
Type: Ginglymus.
Movement: Flexion and extension. The joint is partly extended dorsally in the standing position. Small amount of rotation possible on manipulation.
Bones: Large metacarpal or metatarsal, first phalanx and two proximal sesamoid bones.
Anatomical structures: Joint capsule, two collateral ligamants, nine sesamoidean ligaments, the suspensory ligament. The superficial flexor tendon divides at the level of the fetlock and the deep flexor passes through the ring thus formed. Both tendons are supported by the annular ligament and so give the joint further support.

Conditions
1)   Sprain of the joint or related structures.
2)   DJD.

The fetlock joint (left) *and ligaments* (right)

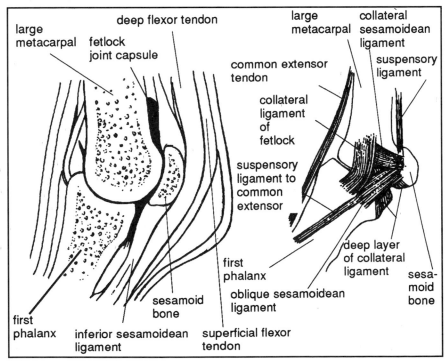

large metacarpal
deep flexor tendon
fetlock joint capsule
large metacarpal
collateral sesamoidean ligament
common extensor tendon
suspensory ligament
collateral ligament of fetlock
suspensory ligament to common extensor
first phalanx
deep layer of collateral ligament
sesamoid bone
oblique sesamoidean ligament
first phalanx
sesamoid bone
inferior sesamoidean ligament
superficial flexor tendon

3)   OCD.
4)   Sesamoiditis.
5)   Flexural deformity of the joint.
6)   Villonodular synovitis.
7)   Articular windgalls.

Conditions of neighbouring structures
1)   Fractures of any of the bones involved.
2)   Epiphysitis.
3)   Bursitis.
4)   Tendon sheath synovitis (tendinous windgalls).

Knee (Carpus)
Type: There are three principle joints in the carpus.
1)   The radiocarpal joint formed between the radius and upper row of
carpal bones.
2)   The intercarpal joint formed between the two rows of carpal
bones.

Ligaments of the knee (carpus)

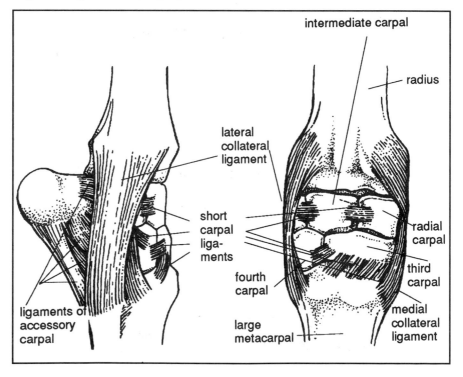

3)   The carpometacarpal joint formed between the lower row of carpal bones and the upper ends of the metacarpal bones.

The first two are ginglymus joints, the last is an arthrodial joint offering virtually no movement. There are also arthrodial joints formed between small bones in the same row of the carpus.

Movement: The principle movement of the whole structure is flexion and extension, though some rotation is possible on manipulation. Virtually all of this movement occurs at the radiocarpal and intercarpal joints.

Bones: There are usually seven carpal bones. The radius above meets the upper row; the lower row meets the upper surfaces of the metacarpal bones.

Anatomical structures: The joint capsule attaches to the extensor tendons in front and forms the front wall of the carpal canal behind; the capsule also continues downward as the inferior check ligament to join the deep flexor tendon in the middle of the cannon area. The synovial membrane forms three sacs corresponding to the three joints with the two lower sacs communicating. There are two collateral ligaments, plus numerous short ligaments between adjacent carpal bones.

Conditions
1)   Sprain of the joint or related structures.
2)   DJD.
3)   Trauma (concussion or bruising), with or without infection.
4)   Developmental deformities.
5)   Fracture.
6)   OCD.

Conditions of neighbouring structures
1)   Carpal tunnel syndrome.
2)   Hygroma of the knee.
3)   Synovitis of the sheaths of the *extensor carpi radialis*, the common and lateral digital extensor tendons.
4)   Epiphysitis of the lower radial growth plate.
5)   Knee splints.
6)   Strain of check ligament.

Elbow Joint
Type: Ginglymus.
Movement: Flexion and extension with some outward movement in extension.
Bones: Humerus, radius and ulna.

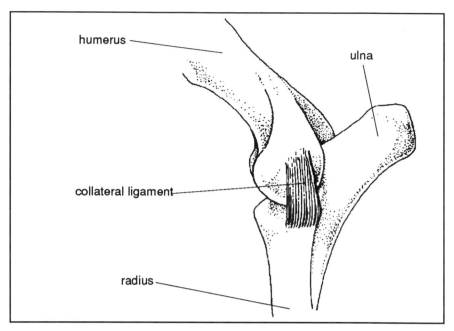

The elbow joint. In addition to the collateral ligament, shown here, there is also ligamentous attachment between the radius and ulna

Anatomical structures: Joint capsule and two collateral ligaments. The radius and ulna are attached by an interosseus ligament which becomes ossified with age and by a transverse ligament, which does not ossify.

Conditions
1)   Sprain of the joint or related structures.
2)   DJD.
3)   OCD.

Conditions of neighbouring structures
1)   Capped elbow.
2)   Fracture of the olecranon.
3)   Separation of the radius and ulna.

Shoulder Joint
Type: Ball-and-socket (enarthrosis).
Movement: Chiefly flexion and extension with some rotation, abduction and adduction.
Bones: Scapula and humerus.
Anatomical structures: Joint capsule. While there are no collateral liga-

ments the muscles in the region provide such strong support that the shoulder joint is seldom dislocated. The intertuberal bursa exists between the front of the humerus and the *biceps brachii* muscle.

Conditions
1)   Sprain of the joint or related structures, including dislocation.
2)   Direct trauma from blows (e.g. hitting gates and doorposts, including fracture).
3)   DJD.
4)   OCD.

Conditions of neighbouring structures
1)   Bicipital bursitis.
2)   Injury to muscles or nerves in the region.

Although there are no lateral ligaments in the shoulder, the joint is adequately supported by muscle surrounding the joint capsule

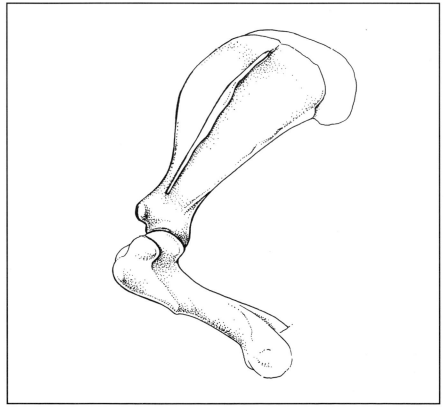

Hind Limb

The coffin, pastern and fetlock joints are similar in detail to those of the forelimb.

Hock (Tarsus)

Type: As in the knee, there are three principle joints in the hock.
1)   Tibiotarsal joint between the tibia and the tibial tarsal bone.
2)   Intertarsal joints between the rows of tarsal bones.
3)   Tarsometatarsal joint between the lower row of tarsal bones and the metatarsals.

The tibiotarsal joint is a ginglymus joint and the principle source of movement in the hock. All other joints between the bones are arthrodial in nature and provide very little movement.
Movement: Mainly flexion and extension.
Bones: Tibia, six tarsal bones and the metatarsals.
Anatomical structures: The joint capsule surrounds the hock and is continued downwards to form the subtarsal check ligament behind. There are

Some ligaments of the hock

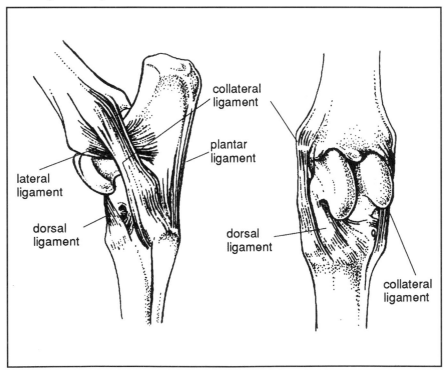

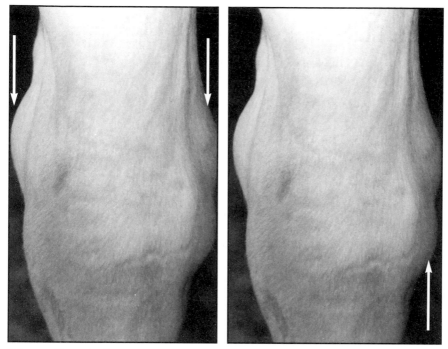

The swellings in bog spavin occur at either side of the joint behind and on the front inner aspect (Photos: Sue Devereux)

four synovial sacs in the hock, the upper two communicating, the lower two do not. There are two lateral and two medial ligaments as well as a dorsal ligament in front and a plantar ligament behind. There are also numerous small ligaments between adjoining bones of the hock.

Conditions
1) Sprain of the joint and related structures (sprung hock).
2) DJD, including bone spavin.
3) OCD.
4) Bog spavin.
5) Developmental deformities.

Conditions of neighbouring structures
1) Curb.
2) Thoroughpin.
3) Capped hock.
4) Displacement of the superficial flexor tendon.
5) Rupture of the Achilles tendon.

Bog spavin is a synovial distension of the true hock joint and occurs generally as a result of trauma, perhaps due to the combined effects of conformation and concussion, and also as a developmental consequence of nutritional problems. In so much as the distension (which is pronounced on the anteromedial and both sides of the back of the hock) is a response to inflammation of the synovial membrane or joint capsule, it must be treated with due concern. If there is lameness, radiographs may be advised. Treatment follows the same lines as recommended for any joint sprain.

The Stifle

Type: The stifle is generally considered collectively as one ginglymus joint, although it is composed of two sub-entities which communicate: the femoropatellar joint and the femorotibial joint. The femoropatellar joint is strictly not a ginglymus joint.

Ligaments of the stifle

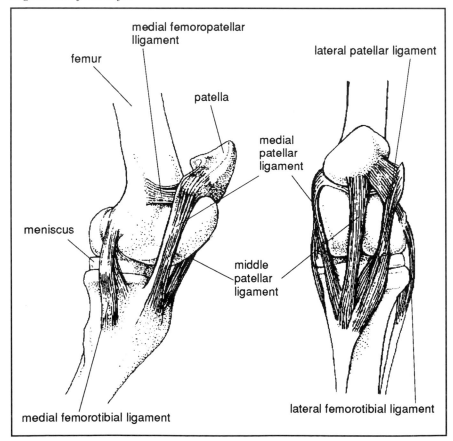

Movment: Mainly flexion and extension.
Bones: The femur, tibia and patella.
Anatomical structures: There are two joint cavities which usually communicate through a slit-like opening. There are two femoropatellar ligaments, lateral and medial, and three patellar ligaments that attach the patella to the front of the tibia.

In the femorotibial joint there are two menisci (discs) which help these bones to articulate with one another (there are consequently two synovial sacs in the femorotibial joint capsule). There are medial, lateral collateral and two cruciate ligaments within the joint itself, situated between the synovial sacs. The lateral ligaments attach the femur to the tibia.

Conditions
1)   Sprain of the joint and related structures.
2)   OCD.
3)   DJD.
4)   Rupture of the cruciate ligaments.
5)   Trauma, with or without infection.
6)   Patellar fixation.
7)   Fracture.

Conditions of neighbouring structures
1)   Subchondral bone cysts (may come into contact with the joint).
2)   Rupture of the muscular support between the pelvis and stifle.

The Hip
Type: Ball-and-socket (enarthrosis).
Movement: Flexion, extension, abduction, adduction and rotation.
Bones: The acetabulum of the pelvis and the femur.
Anatomical structures: Joint capsule, round ligament, accessory ligament.
The accessory ligament limits abduction of the limb.

Conditions
1)   Sprain of the joint and related structures, including dislocation.
2)   OCD.
3)   DJD.
4)   Rupture of the round ligament.

Conditions of neighbouring structures
1)   Fractures involving the pelvis and/or acetabulum.
2)   Muscular injuries over the hip.

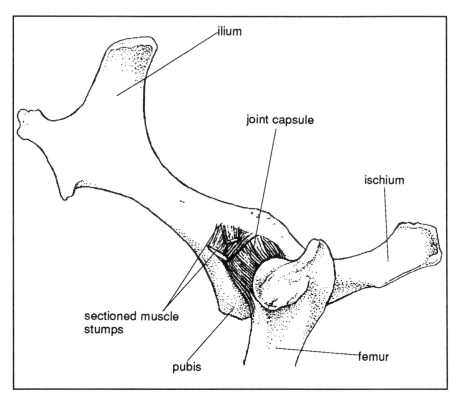

Ligaments of the hip joint

Sacroiliac Joint
Type: Diarthroidal.
Movement: Almost no movement. The purpose of this joint is to form a stable union between the bones involved.
Bones: Sacrum and ilium.
Anatomical structures: Joint capsule, fibrous union and sacroiliac ligament.

Conditions
1)   Sprain of the joint and related structures.
2)   Subluxation (momentary or partial dislocation).

Conditions of neighbouring structures
1)   Injury of surrounding muscles.
2)   Injury of adjacent spinal structures.
Lameness related to sacroiliac joint disease is diagnosed on the basis of anatomical changes which develop because the union between sacrum

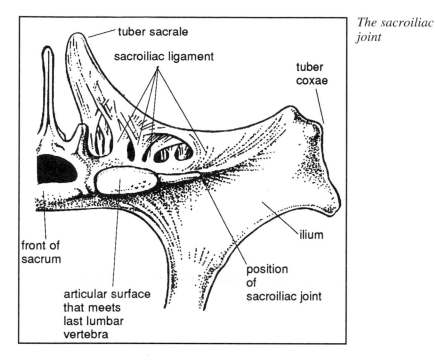

The sacroiliac joint

and ilium is disrupted. There is usually muscle wastage on the affected side together with pain on manipulation of the overlying area.

Treatment involves manipulation followed by laser or ultrasound therapy to relieve pain and inflammation, and Faradic-type stimulation to restore normal muscle use.

Luxation

Luxation, or dislocation, of a joint occurs when there is serious trauma to the supporting structures resulting in displacement of the bones forming the joint. It is extremely serious and requires immediate reduction (replacement of normal anatomy) of the bones together with strong support, where possible, and the use of pain-killing and anti-inflammatory drugs.

Subluxation

Subluxation is the term used to describe an injury where the bony constituents of a joint momentarily lose their correct relationships but return at once to the normal state. This inevitably stretches the supporting tissues.

8 The Nervous and Muscular Systems

All movement occurs under control from the nervous system. However, it is contraction of muscle that effects movement by acting through bones and joints.

The Vertebral Column

The skull and vertebral column are the bony protection for the brain and spinal cord, the nervous system that controls virtually all activity within the body. The vertebrae are divided according to their situation in the column and have characteristic differences which relate to the functional requirements of each area. They all consist of three basic parts: a body, an arch and processes.

The divisions are as follows.

Cervical Vertebrae

There are seven cervical vertebrae, the first two of which, the atlas and axis respectively, differ from the rest. The atlas has no body, being simply a short ring or tube on either side of which is a large wing. The whole bone is a similar shape to a tortoise shell. The atlas articulates in front with the skull. The axis has at its front the tooth-like odontoid process that extends forwards into the lower part of the ring in the atlas, thus providing a structure about which the atlas can rotate. The axis also possesses a strong dorsal spinous process which gives attachment to part of the *ligamentum nuchae*, the ligament that runs from the withers to the nuchal crest of the

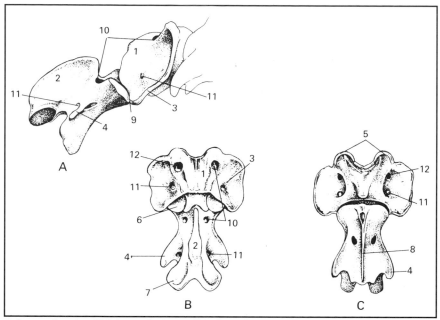

Atlas and axis: (A) lateral view; (B) dorsal view; (C) ventral view. (1) dorsal arch of atlas; (2) spinous process of axis; (3) wing of atlas; (4) transverse process of axis; (5) anterior articular cavities of atlas; (6) anterior articular process of axis; (7) posterior articular process of axis; (8) ventral spine of axis; (9) odontoid process of axis; (10) intervertebral foramina; (11) transverse foramina; (12) alar foramen

occiput of the skull, and that supports the head and neck. Each of the rest of the cervical vertebrae is composed of a body surmounted by an arch on top of which is a low dorsal spinous process; there are also transverse processes which are prominent and plate-like and can be felt under the skin of the neck.

Thoracic Vertebrae

There are 18 thoracic vertebrae, between each pair of which a rib is situated. The bodies are shorter than those of the cervical vertebrae but the dorsal spines are particularly high (these are at their highest in the withers region). The transverse processes are relatively short.

Lumbar Vertebrae

There are usually six lumbar vertebrae (occasionally five). In these, the transverse processes are long and wide, providing spinal support in the

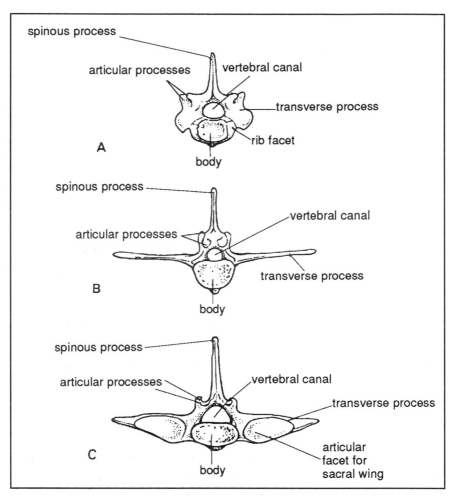

Vertebrae in posterior view: (A) *first thoracic;* (B) *first lumbar;* (C) *last lumbar*

region between the last rib and the sacrum (at the front of the pelvis). The last three lumbar vertebrae have articular facets on the lateral processes, forming synovial joints that tend to become calcified with age (sometimes beginning as early as two years). The dorsal spines are similar in length to those of the more posterior thoracic spines.

The Sacrum

The sacrum consists of five bones (vertebrae) which are fused from an early age. It is triangular in form and lies on the roof of the pelvic cavity with its posterior end a little higher than its front. The pelvic bones are

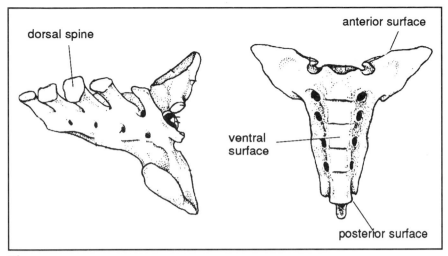

The sacrum

united with the sacrum through the ilia at the sacroiliac joints. The dorsal spines diminish in height from front to back. The lumbosacral articulation consists of one central and two lateral synovial joints that persist in function throughout life as a rule. Although the vertebral column has limited movement in the whole thoracic/lumbar/sacral region, there is a certain amount of flexion and extension in locomotion.

Coccygeal Vertebrae

There are 18 coccygeal vertebrae, the last of which are short rods united by discs of cartilage.

Between the bodies of each two vertebrae there is a cartilaginous disc. All vertebrae are bound by dorsal, ventral and lateral ligaments, by joint capsules and by the supraspinous ligament that runs from the skull to the sacrum and which, in the neck, forms the *ligamentum nuchae*.

A total of 42 pairs of spinal nerves emerge from between adjacent vertebrae and these ultimately supply all voluntary muscle and skin. They are the means through which an animal perceives external stimuli (e.g. heat, cold, trauma) and responds to them (circulatory changes or movement).

The Voluntary Nervous System

The voluntary nervous system is that which allows an animal to move and relate to its environment. Being under voluntary control, each muscle has

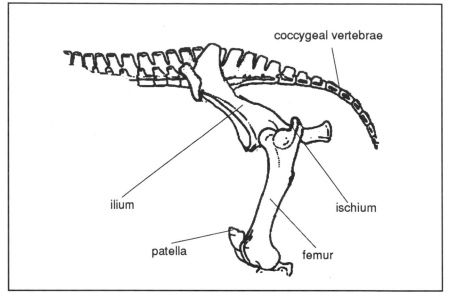

The coccygeal vertebrae are the bones of the tail

a voluntary nerve supply. This system provides control of the complex movements of ambulation, of taking flight, of evasion, or other action. Nerves can be mechanically injured; paralysis is the common result of this, as is seen in the shoulder and forearm after injury to the radial nerve. Similar injuries may affect nerves in any exposed area of the body.

Reflex Arcs

The nervous system operates extensively through the presence of reflexes (involuntary responses) which are controlled by simple reflex arcs. These are neural paths along which impulses travel to produce a reflex action, and they allow for many different types of reaction to external stimuli (e.g. when an injection needle is pricked into the leg of an animal that is not being restrained; the immediate withdrawal of the limb is a reflex action, done without thought, a spontaneous consequence of the insult).

This action operates through means of a reflex arc. The animal may then decide to kick, but this is now a voluntary act, operating directly under the central control of the brain.

Other reflex arcs are more complex than this (e.g. sensory nerve endings exist in muscle which are triggered by contraction and relaxation). Thus, contraction in one leg might result in relaxation of a muscle in another. Note how, at the walk, one forelimb is contracting and being protracted as the other is weight bearing and in extension. One of these

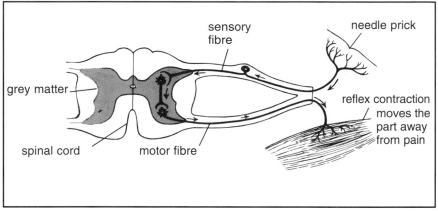

The reflex arc

actions stimulates an opposing reaction at the other end of a reflex arc. While a certain amount of this movement is within voluntary control, a great deal is reflex, but still under the control of higher centres in the brain which have the ability to override local reflexes. These higher centres will decide on avoiding action, when needed, or decide when it is necessary to pull up. There would be very little movement if every individual action had to be thought about first, so reflexes are important. However, there is always the overriding influence of voluntary control, watching, listening and the ability to react. We see the functioning of reflexes as a normal part of ambulation and only detect their loss as a failure of movement or coordination. Yet this failure may well be an indication of injury or disease in the nervous system and so has its importance here.

Natural Conformational Deviations of the Back

Roach back is a natural conformation of the back in which the dorsal spines of the more posterior thoracic vertebrae and the lumbar region have a marked convexity in lateral profile. It is not an unsoundness and is not a symptom of any inherent abnormality. Dipped back is also conformational; in exaggerated cases it amounts to weakness and is likely to lead to lameness at some stage.

Lameness of Spinal Origin

Within professional circles there has always been discussion about the sig-

significance of spinal structures in lameness. Knowledge of this area is evolving rapidly.

Definition
Lameness of spinal origin occurs in all types of horses but is especially prevalent in those that compete actively, and particularly those that jump. The problem arises from minor movements of adjacent spinal structures leading to muscle spasm and pain which may reflect pressure on emerging spinal nerves.

Causes
The most common cause of the condition is uncoordinated or violent movement, especially when jumping. This occurs because the natural inclination of the thoracic/lumbar/sacral parts of the spine is to maintain a rigid attitude that protects the spinal cord from potential trauma at times of greatest risk (fast gaits and when jumping).

However, the forces involved in locomotion are favoured by ventral flexion of the spine to allow for greater extension of the limbs, and dorsiflexion can occur naturally at the point of landing or take-off, but if either of these movements is excessive it can result in injury. These unwelcome influences on spinal integrity may be further added to by the weight of a rider.

Signs
These vary with the part of the spine and the vertebrae affected. Lameness may be marked, or the action of the horse may only be marginally altered.

Lameness of spinal origin is usually represented by a swinging-leg lameness in which length and direction of stride are most likely to be affected. The horse may not be nodding when the limb strikes the ground though movement is perceptibly altered. It is not unusual for two limbs on one diagonal to be moving abnormally.

Diagnosis and location of the lesion is based on observation and manipulation of the spinal column. If the problem exists in the cervical region, an affected horse may tend to favour one side, and lateral bending of the head and neck is often more difficult to achieve on one side than the other. There may be pain on surface manipulation and spasm may be noted in cervical muscles.

If the problem exists in the thoracic/lumbar/sacral region, pain is usually evident on surface manipulation. Muscle spasm may create minor distortions of the superficial outline of the bones in particularly aggravated cases. Muscle atrophy may occur from lack of use, further exaggerating the physical distortion. Primary muscle injury can also occur at the time of the initial injury and this can result in swelling rather than atrophy.

Treatment
Manipulation effectively restores full movement to affected areas in a significant percentage of cases where there is no serious disruption of spinal structures. Any muscular injury related to the problem is treated separately. Some animals are predisposed to this kind of lameness and are manipulated routinely as a preventive. Many good horses have back problems which seriously affect their performances, but are controlled by constant vigilance and preventive care.

Other Neurological Problems

We have looked at general neurological problems already; now we look at some specific clinical entities of nervous origin.

Wobbler (Cervical Vertebral Malformation)

While this condition has been recognised for many years, an understanding of its pathology is more recent.

Definition
A wobbler is a horse suffering from posterior incoordination. There is loose action that is not natural and which is outside voluntary control.

Causes
The condition is generally considered to be due to spinal cord compression in the neck region. This may be developmental or may be as a consequence of trauma. It usually occurs in young horses of all breeds and is thought to be most common in Thoroughbreds. The strongly developing animal appears most at risk. It can also occur in older horses.

Signs
The onset of the condition is sudden. The most common sign is disjointed movement in the hind limbs and an apparent inability to place the feet properly when asked to turn sharply or reverse. As the condition represents pressure on the spinal cord, nervous control of movement is abnormal. Voluntary movements are impeded and the animal displays this clearly. There may be a tendency to fall. The condition is usually pro-

gressive and the forelimbs are often affected later than the hind limbs.

Treatment
The condition is incurable although some horses may survive for breeding purposes; however, as there is a suggestion that the disease is hereditary, this is probably unwise. There is also a body of opinion that aligns the condition with OCD (in which case it is likely to be developmental).

A similar condition is known to exist in Arabs and Morgans and occurs usually in the first year of life.

Shivering

The title of this condition reflects the symptoms of disease and does not relate to the conventional meaning of the word.

Definition
This is a condition of unknown cause in which the affected horse has a characteristic action of the hind limbs and tail which are effectively described by the name. A loss of voluntary control suggests the disease is of nervous origin.

Signs
A horse may show signs of shivering in normal forward movement when a limb is lifted and held involuntarily with a marked quivering action. It may be encouraged to display this when asked to move backwards, when

When backed, a shiverer shows involuntary movement of the tail

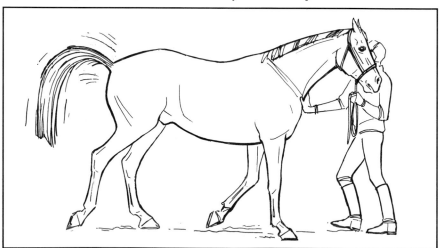

the tail is also lifted and seen to shake in a repeated, spasmodic way. The animal might also have difficulty in placing its feet when asked to turn sharply.

Treatment
Although the condition is incurable, mildly affected horses may be safe to ride, but would never be passed sound for sales purposes.

Stringhalt

Again, in this condition the common term describes the symptoms of the disease, which are easily recognised.

Definition
The hind limbs are lifted excessively in movement and the horse displays a clear involuntary snatching action in its affected limbs. The cause of the condition is unknown although the symptoms suggest it is of nervous origin.

Signs
One or both hind limbs may be affected. The limb is lifted from the ground as the horse moves forward and appears to shudder during protraction.

First steps may be exaggerated before the horse finds its stride. Varying degrees of abnormality are seen and early signs may be slight. The symp-

Movement in stringhalt is involuntary and usually seen as the horse moves off

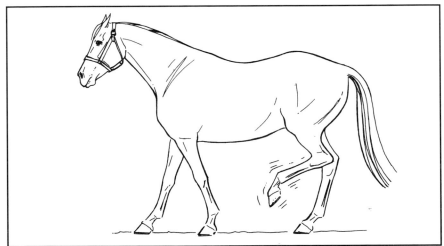

toms are generally confined to the action of the limb as opposed to shivering where more central nervous involvement is suggested.

Treatment
Surgery involves removing part of the lateral digital extensor tendon, and is performed with some degree of success. The condition can be progressive although some horses remain functionally sound and can even race.

Australian stringhalt is a more pronounced condition with the same clinical symptoms. It is thought to be caused by an ingested plant toxin and affected animals generally recover.

Dropped Elbow (Radial paralysis)

While conditions involving nerve injury can occur in any area with a nerve supply, certain areas are most commonly involved and certain disease entities specifically recognised.

Definition
This condition is the result of injury to the radial nerve in the region of the shoulder. The radial nerve supplies the muscles which extend the elbow, knee and foot. Paralysis of these muscles therefore results in partial limb flexion with the inability to extend.

Causes
It usually occurs from a direct blow, perhaps in a fall, or by running into a hard object like a wall or fence. The injury occurs most commonly where the nerve crosses the humerus. It may also be caused by an injury in the region of the first rib.

Signs
The signs of this condition are easily recognised. Typically, the elbow drops from its natural position and the limb is held flexed (or flaccid), the animal generally being unable to bring it forward. No weight is borne on the affected limb and the foot may be dragged along the ground if the animal is able to move. Paralysis is reflected in restricted (or lost) movement and there may be no feeling below the area of the initial injury.

Treatment
Physiotherapy aims to heal the damaged tissues and restore function to paralysed muscles. While complete severing of the nerve would present a hopeless prognosis, many of these cases are returned to normal with prop-

er care. Repair of nervous tissues is slow but the eventual result in most cases is well worth the time and patience. However, it should be appreciated, that Faradic stimulation of muscle is not effective where the nerve supply to the muscle has been cut off through injury. This is because muscle contraction is dependent on the integrity of its nerve supply.

Crural Nerve Paralysis

Crural nerve paralysis is a similar condition in the hind limb caused by injury to the nerve that supplies the large muscle mass (the *quadriceps femoris*) which is inserted into the patella. The limb is held flexed in the standing position (though there may be flaccid lengthening of the muscles above the stifle at the front of the limb) and extension is impaired, though not completely lost. The condition may be confused with rupture of the *quadriceps femoris* in which symptoms are similar, or of the *tensor fascia lata* which connects the tuber coxae of the ilium with the patella.

Treatment follows the same lines as for dropped elbow.

Sweeny

Sweeny (suprascapular paralysis) is also sometimes called 'dropped shoulder'.

Definition
This describes atrophy of the *supraspinatus* and *infraspinatus* muscles that cover the scapula. The name is also sometimes applied to muscle atrophy in other areas.

Causes
Sweeny is caused by injury to the suprascapular nerve that supplies these muscles. It may occur as a result of a fall or from striking solid objects such as a door post.

Signs
The shoulder area in established cases is shrunken and flattened with abnormal prominence of the joint and the scapular spine. The signs are so typical that diagnosis is obvious.

Treatment
This is the same as for radial paralysis. Electrical stimulation may help reintroduce muscle tone, when the nerve has repaired. However, this can

be extremely slow and some cases never recover fully. The nerve must be allowed to recover first, then muscle stimulation may bring back full muscle use.

The Muscular System

Skeletal muscle is muscle which is under voluntary control; it includes all the muscles involved in locomotion, the normal function of which is flexion, extension, abduction or adduction. Each muscle body consists of bundles of fibres whose functional effect is achieved through contraction and relaxation. Many skeletal muscles are attached to bone at either end, and the effect of contraction on an intervening structure (perhaps a joint) is to create movement. Some muscles (such as the limb flexors) have tendons of varying length which are continuous with the muscle body. Consequently, these muscles are attached to bones which are remote from one another: the deep flexor of the forelimb has a muscular attachment on the humerus and the far end of the tendon is inserted onto the most distant limb bone, the third phalanx. Thus it influences all intervening joints when in use.

Flexors have their influence on the back of the limb which they take from the ground and raise so that it can then be moved forward for the next phase of the stride.

Limb extensor muscles are situated at the front of the limb and are responsible for forward placement (protraction).

Adductors and abductors move the limb towards or away from a straight-bearing plane, respectively.

Muscles may act in unison with one another, in which case they are described as synergistic. Those that have opposite actions are antagonistic.

Each muscle has an abundant blood supply, because the act of contraction is dependent on a continuous energy and oxygen supply under normal circumstances. Most slow-pace exercise is termed aerobic, because the supply of oxygen through respiration is adequate to supply its needs. Anaerobic muscle contraction occurs at sprinting pace, when the circulating blood is unable to provide the oxygen required; this is then provided by oxygen bound to the myoglobin molecule within the muscle cell itself.

Each muscle is provided with a voluntary nerve supply which allows it to work under voluntary control. There is also an extensive system of local reflexes which allows for a great deal of movement to be conducted automatically.

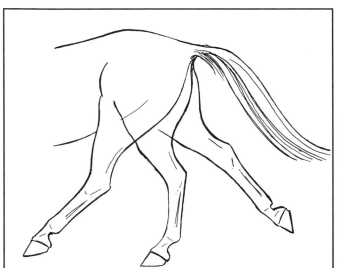

The hind limb in forward extension (left), *support* (centre) *and backward extension* (right). *Backward extension is followed by flexion to bring the limb forward to forward extension*

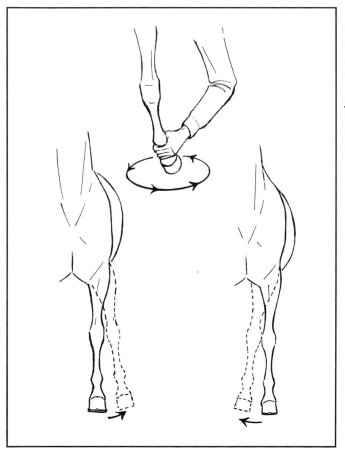

Passive rotation (top) *with the limb off the ground. Abduction* (left) *away from the centre line. Adduction* (right) *towards the centre line*

Voluntary Muscle Types

Three main types of fibre have been identified in equine skeletal muscle - distinct from cardiac muscle (found only in the heart) and smooth muscle (which is located in organs such as the bowel) - and they are designated as Type 1, Type 2a, and Type 2b. It is thought that athletic ability is related to the distribution of different fibre types in an animal's muscle.

Type 1 fibres are slow-twitch red fibres which have a slow speed of contraction. They exhibit little fatigue and animals with a predominance of Type 1 fibres are likely to be best in endurance events.

Type 2a fibres are fast-twitch white fibres which fatigue easily. These are used for short powerful bursts of activity.

Type 2b fibres are fast-twitch white (high-oxidative) fibres, which resist fatigue better than Type 2a fibres and are used for more sustained activity.

All three fibre types exist within the same muscle body and the relative proportions of each decide performance type (e.g. sprinter, stayer, etc.).

Muscular Injury

Muscular injury is largely neglected as a source of lameness, a situation that needs serious reappraisal.

Primary Muscle Injury (or Strain)

The term 'primary muscle injury' is used here to denote a kind of injury common in horses that is similar to the type of muscular injury suffered by human athletes.

It is not uncommon for the muscle fibres of athletic animals to be torn or ruptured during exercise. This occurs as commonly in horses as it does in human athletes and the extent varies from small groups of fibres to whole muscle bodies. It is followed by haemorrhage, then formation of a clot. The functional effect of this is that the affected muscle is taken out of use by the body (as a result of pain) and effort is made to compensate for its loss by recruitment of other muscle groups during movement. This inevitably leads to an alteration of action (however slight). The consequence to the limb may result in secondary injury because of abnormal foot placement or weight distribution.

Muscular injuries are divided into two types: primary injury - by far the most common, due to uncomplicated muscle fibre rupture; and secondary muscle damage - usually associated with underlying bony disturbance. The latter is an important consideration because it is not uncommon to find fractures associated with gross muscular damage in areas such as the pelvis.

Atrophy is a feature of chronic muscular injury, and is particularly seen in the shoulder and upper pelvic areas as flat or shrunken muscle (e.g. as in sweeny). It is caused by a decrease in volume of an unused muscle after injury, or sometimes when its nerve supply has been directly interfered with by trauma. Atrophy will occur more generally when an area is immobilised (e.g. after the application of a cast) and it is also sometimes seen as an expression of malnutrition and senility.

Causes

It is recognised that the size and strength of muscle fibres increase with training, therefore the greatest incidence of muscular injury occurs when these are less than fully strengthened. Injuries occur typically when a horse is being exercised and may be related to sudden explosive changes of pace, such as when breaking into a gallop, when quickening, or even when jumping. There is a possibility the injury might indicate fatigue in a muscle that is not adequately fit for the work it is being subjected to.

Imbalance of muscular coordination can also cause injury, even fracture, when the pull of opposing muscle groups is out of synchronisation. This can arise when a horse plunges or tries to save itself when it slips, or when an animal is recumbent and recovering from anaesthesia. Injury may occur, too, when a limb suddenly has to be projected forwards in order to prevent a fall, or through direct trauma such as a kick.

Signs

Tearing occurs more often in the larger muscle bodies, therefore injuries are common in the neck, shoulders, back, quarters and thighs, but they are less common in the gaskin and forearm.

Muscular lameness is often ignored because it soon passes off. Thus an injury to the long head of the *triceps brachii* (between the scapula and elbow), for example, results in the forelimb being used in a way that avoids or reduces the effective working of this muscle. The result is a change in limb action, often without overt lameness, that may be barely detectable. The straight extension/flexion process may be altered to a movement that may exhibit some abduction or rotation. If only a small segment of muscle has ruptured, the dynamic effect of the injury may be minimal. In any case, the effect is to shorten the potential stretch of the muscle, or muscle fibres, involved. The affected muscle is thus held as if

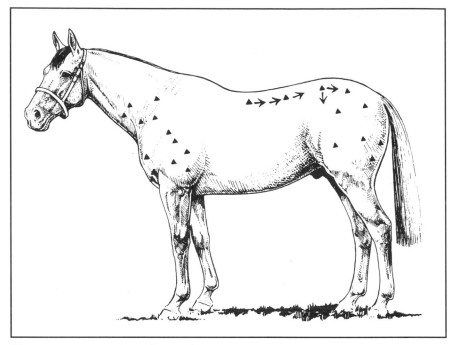

The most common sites of muscular injury

partially contracted; the influence of this on limb dynamics is (with the forelimb) to place a greater strain on the less elastic tendons. It may also cause deviation in protraction in a manner that interferes with proper placement of the foot on the ground.

The horse is lame immediately after tearing a muscle but this passes off with time, and other muscles in the limb compensate and take over its functions. As a result, these other muscles are sometimes over-loaded and subsequently suffer injury. There is swelling of the injured area but damage is best detected by the use of a Faradic-type electrical muscle stimulating equipment, which is both diagnostic and therapeutic. Muscular injuries seldom cure themselves, and an animal may have a permanently altered action if the condition is not treated.

The initial lameness, when there is evident pain and a marked supporting-leg lameness, does not usually last for more than a day or two. However, there is lameness in movement, the action of the limb being inhibited at the trot (and faster gaits).

Injury to muscles of the loins, quarters and neck, however, may account for longer-lasting initial lameness. Diagnosis of muscular injury is possible using ultrasonic scanning, muscle biopsy, and blood tests. However, a quick and specific diagnosis is possible through clinical means.

Treatment

The modern way to monitor muscle health and treat injuries is with forms of physical therapy that include muscle stimulation with Faradic-type equipment. The method, diagnostic as well as curative, promotes organisation and repair of damaged tissues and the forced return of injured muscle into work.

This treatment is accompanied by controlled exercise which encourages re-use of muscle in a manner that limits the risk of further injury. It is important that this be continued until the animal's action is fully restored. It is far from certain, contrary to common belief, that muscular injuries will correct themselves without treatment. In fact, the reverse is more generally true; and where cartilage and bone formation is found in muscle it is most probably preceded by simple primary injuries which were not effectively treated (with the exception of the congenital condition described in foals).

An extensive range of equipment is now marketed for muscle treatment. However, some of the treatments only relieve pain and stimulate circulation of the injured part, their effect being palliative and short term. The injury is unlikely to be cured unless damaged tissues are encouraged to return to effective use.

When muscle injury accompanies bone damage (e.g. as in pelvic fractures) treatment of the muscular problem may not be advisable initially. It may in fact adversely influence the condition and allow greater displacement of the broken bone ends. However, when the bone has repaired (as is common in the pelvis), the muscle may then require stimulation to restore full use to the part.

Fibrotic Myopathy

Myopathy being disease of muscle, fibrotic myopathy describes fibrous tissue, cartilage and bone formation within muscle.

Definition

This term is used to describe injuries which occur in *semitendinosus, semimembranosus* and *biceps femoris* muscles of the hind limb. Fibrotic myopathy, although most commonly identified in this region could easily occur in any region of chronic muscle injury.

Causes

Although the condition has been identified in newborn foals, in the adult it is usually a consequence of earlier muscle strain. Despite the initial injury the animal will have remained in exercise and while there may be repeated bouts of lameness when the injury has been aggravated there is generally no intensive effort to treat it (except perhaps with drugs).

Signs

There is usually a gross distortion of the anatomy of the area with palpable hard swellings in the muscle bodies. There may be slight upward pulling on the hock, creating the impression of the animal being straighter in the affected limb. The stride on the affected side is shortened and the limb, after being fully protracted, may be retracted before foot placement occurs.

Diagnosis is easily confirmed through muscle stimulation.

Treatment

The treatment is the same as for primary muscle injury, although it will take a considerable time to restore full use of the affected muscles. If the condition is too far advanced, it may not be possible to reverse it except by surgery. However, even after surgical correction, it is unlikely that an affected limb can be restored to full normal action.

Prevention demands early diagnosis of muscle injury and timely treatment to avoid this condition.

Rupture of the Peroneus Tertius Muscle

While only a few specific muscle injuries are specified in veterinary literature, any muscle body can be ruptured. The condition described here is noteworthy because of its particular symptoms.

Definition

This muscle is part of the reciprocal apparatus of the hind limb. It effectively prevents the hock or stifle flexing independently of one another. The *peroneus tertius* is mostly tendinous in nature, it originates from the lower end of the femur, and is inserted onto the upper end of the large metatarsal bone (cannon).

Causes

Rupture occurs as a result of sudden explosive movement or through violent effort (e.g. when a limb is caught in a fence or ditch).

Signs
The most characteristic sign is the ability of the animal to flex the stifle independently of the hock. There is marked lameness and on lifting the leg and extending it backwards there is evident dimpling of the Achilles tendon above the hock, which cannot occur normally.

Treatment
Complete box rest is indicated for a period of not less than four weeks, and the horse is reintroduced to work slowly. The prognosis is guarded.

Rupture of the Gastrocnemius Muscle

As opposed to the *peroneus tertius*, the *gastrocnemius* consists of a fleshy muscle which has a tendon attached to it.

Definition
The *gastrocnemius* muscle is attached to the point of the hock through the Achilles tendon. The Achilles tendon is composed of the *gastrocnemius* and superficial flexor tendons combined.

Causes
Excessive extension of the hock.

Signs
The hock, having lost the support of the Achilles tendon, drops backwards out of position and the hock seems overbent when compared with its fellow. The condition can occur in both limbs at the same time. If the rupture is partial, the horse will still be able to use the limb, though its action will be abnormal. If the rupture is complete (involving the full Achilles tendon), the limb will be unable to bear weight.

Treatment
As the weight of the animal tends to draw the torn ends apart any hope of repair depends on nullifying this effect and promoting natural tissue repair with laser or ultrasound therapy.
 The prognosis is not good because of the tendency for natural limb dynamics to draw the injured ends apart.

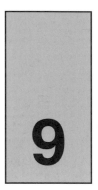

9 Other Lamenesses

Conditions described in this chapter do not readily lend themselves to any of the classifications already considered.

Upward Fixation of the Patella

The patella is regarded to be a large sesamoid bone that develops in the tendon of the quadriceps femoris muscle. The purpose of a sesamoid bone is to give mechanical advantage to muscles by providing added leverage.

Definition
The condition is marked by locking of the patella (the bone that corresponds to the human kneecap) on the inner trochlear ridge of the femur. This is the normal position the patella adopts when the horse is resting and the stay apparatus is engaged. However, it is not a position which is compatible with normal locomotion. The patella is naturally seated in a groove at the end of the femur and is held in position by a number of ligaments. In upward fixation it slips out of the groove onto the medial ridge and is held there, stretching the ligaments. Once this has happened, the stretched ligaments make it more likely to happen again. It may occur in only one hind leg, but it is common for both limbs to be affected in time.

Causes
This is often thought to have an hereditary predisposition, but it occurs in a number of different circumstances. It is more likely to happen in legs with an upright stifle. Poor physical condition seems to make an animal

susceptible to it, and upward fixation may also be precipitated by sharp work up steep inclines in predisposed horses.

Signs
The leg is locked in extension and the horse will generally refuse to bear weight on the affected limb when fixation occurs. The stifle and hock cannot flex, but the fetlock can. The locking may last for hours or only moments. In some cases it keeps locking and releasing itself. If the horse is forced to move it will drag the affected foot along the ground. A typical sharp crack or clicking sound may be heard when the patella is released.

Sometimes locking occurs as the animal begins to move off and the patella is quickly released again with a similar characteristic clicking noise.

The symptom of rigid extension of a hind leg is typical, and the problem is not relieved until the animal manages to free the fixed patella - possibly by a sudden movement. The condition can occur in animals of all ages from yearling upwards.

Treatment
By putting a sideline (i.e. a rope attached to the fetlock and looped around the neck) on the affected limb and lifting it forward towards the neck, the patella may be released. Direct pressure on the patella itself may help return it to its natural position, especially if the effort aims to lift it upwards and laterally.

The bedding for affected horses should be of paper or shavings to help the animal get around the stable with ease.

Anti-inflammatory drugs will help keep any reaction within the stifle to a minimum but will have no long-term effect on the condition.

Surgery is performed on older horses with a history of a recurrent problem, involving section of the medial patellar ligament. The results of the operation are good although complications occur in a percentage of cases suggesting that the operation should only be undertaken with a good deal of consideration.

Luxation of the Patella

Luxation of the patella is a different congenital condition from that of upward fixation.

It features displacement of the patella either laterally or medially due to conformational abnormality of the femoral condyles. Surgery, aimed at stabilising the patella, may be succcessful in some cases.

Filling in the Legs

There is no special clinical term to describe this condition, which is a normal feature of horse management.

Definition
This term 'filling in the legs' is used to describe the passive filling of the legs of stabled horses in which there are varying degrees of uniform swelling with obliteration of the normal anatomical outlines. It occurs as an expression of circulatory stagnation and is mainly a benign condition that disappears with exercise.

Blood fluids are retained in the limbs instead of being returned to the general circulation.

Causes
While the legs of horses confined to their boxes are likely to fill through lack of exercise, the condition is more commonly related to mild toxic conditions stemming from the bowel, or, similarly, digestive upsets. It can also occur as a consequence of feed change or as a result of over-feeding. Filling may appear as an expression of circulatory disease. It is also a common feature of equine viral arteritis (EVA).

Signs
Filling is generally noted in the morning and may disappear with exercise. A single occurrence might not be noteworthy but, with competing animals, may be accompanied by a reduction in the level of performance.

A critical factor is that filling is noted in more than one limb, very often all four. When only one limb is filled it is wise to consider an alternative cause, such as infection.

Treatment
Laxatives or purgatives may be necessary to relieve the symptoms, but should not be used to excess. The horse is then returned to a simple diet of hay and small quantities of oats.

Horses whose legs fill when fed on heavy concentrate diets should have the quantity reduced or the feed changed.

Most legs fill after injuries and this distinct type of filling is associated with wounds and grazes. The cause is interference with normal limb circulation. This type of filling takes longer to disappear, but need not always keep an animal out of work.

Where circulation is a cause of filling, the situation is more serious and professional advice is needed to determine the soundness of the heart and other organs.

Lymphangitis

The term 'lymphangitis' applies to a condition marked by extensive filling of, usually, one hind leg.

Definition
Lymphangitis is defined as inflammation of a lymphatic vessel. The lymphatic system exists on the venous side of the circulation and carries lymph into the venous system and liver from the extremities and bowel. The lymph glands are set along the course of these veins and vessels, and their purpose is to filter off foreign material, including organisms, and prevent them from getting deeper into the body.

Filling involves the lymphatic vessels and glands. The whole leg may be swollen from the ground to stifle or elbow.

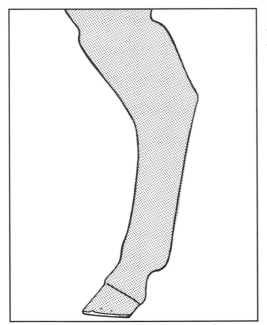

The swelling in lymphangitis obliterates normal limb anatomy

Causes
Lymphangitis occurs most commonly in housed animals on hard feed, suggesting a dietary cause. It may also be precipitated by trauma or infection.

Signs
Swelling is extensive and the limb may appear stretched to capacity. The skin may even weep in severe cases. There is usually localised pain on the course of the leg lymphatic vessels. The animal may sweat and have a raised temperature. Lameness of the affected limb is marked.

Diagnosis is based on the nature and size of the swelling and the condition must not be confused with physical injuries.

Treatment
Antihistamine and anti-inflammatory drugs are used to control the tissue rections which lead to the condition. In some cases the response is quick. Laxative diets and purgatives may help, as may diuretics. It is important to encourage the animal to use the affected limb in order to assist circulation.

The limb may retain permanent signs of the problem and recurring episodes are common in individual cases; each of these may leave the leg a little larger. Horses which have suffered one attack should be exercised regularly and lightly lunged on rest days.

Hereditary Multiple Exostosis

This is a rare condition, marked by irregular swellings on the bones of the limbs, ribs and pelvis. The swellings, which are recognised as distortions of normal anatomy, may interfere with the function of other structures, depending on their positioning and so cause lameness.

There is no known treatment and affected animals should not be used for breeding purposes.

Marie's Disease

Marie's disease (hypertrophic pulmonary osteoarthropathy) received a recent notoriety owing to its diagnosis in a leading Thoroughbred stallion.

It is marked by irregular enlargements in the long bones of the limbs and is thought to be associated with lung tumours and tuberculosis.

Affected animals are given a poor prognosis. However, the above mentioned stallion survived and many other animals affected with this condition have done likewise, suggesting that there may be other causes. Many continue to live normal lives without any need for ongoing treatment.

Osteomyelitis

Osteomyelitis is the infection of bone and it can occur as the consequence of deep penetrating wounds bringing the infective source to the bone, or as a blood-borne disease of foals.

Intensive antibiotic treatment is indicated together with proper wound cleansing and the removal of foreign matter and contaminating material.

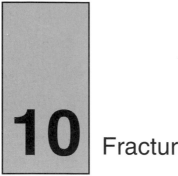

10 Fractures

Bone fractures occur as a result of direct trauma and are classified as simple fractures if there are just two pieces, and compound fractures if the skin is broken.

With communited fractures the bone is broken into more than two pieces, and with incomplete fractures the whole substance of the bone is

Fractures of the limb: (top row, from left) *simple fracture without displacement; with displacement; and a communited fracture;* (bottom row, from left) *compound fracture with the skin broken; articular fracture, involving a joint; and incomplete fracture, not penetrating the full depth of the bone*

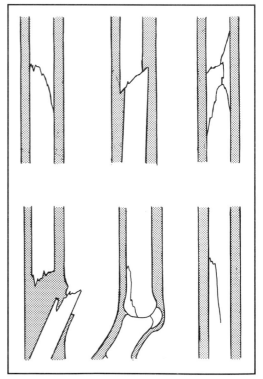

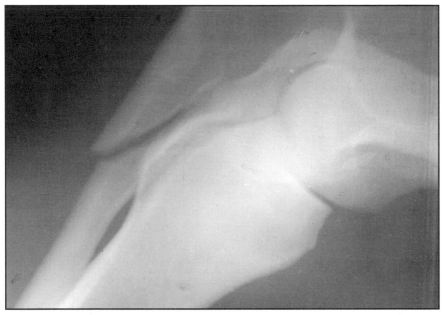

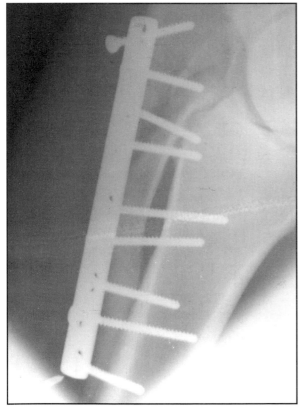

Radiograph (above) *of a fracture of the ulna;* (left) *the same fracture plated*

Radiograph showing fracture of the third carpal bone

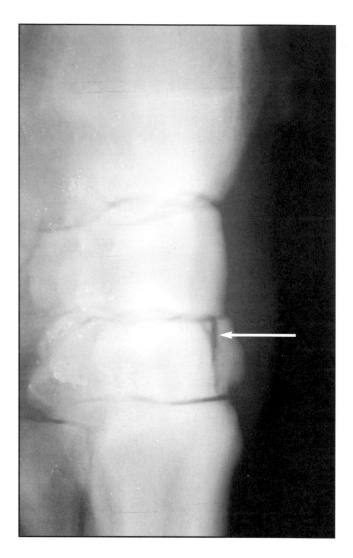

not penetrated and the bone does not separate. When the ends of the fractured bone are not in apposition the term used is 'displaced' and these ends will need to be replaced if the fracture is to heal satisfactorily.

Fractures that traverse a joint are articular fractures. A common complication of articular fractures is DJD.

The repair of large bones is limited by the nature of the horse and the difficulties imposed by the mechanics of bone healing. Temperamentally, most horses are not disposed to being held in slings while their bones mend, and the physical limitations of bone repair mean the parts must be immobilised and free of weight if the repair is to be a success. However, modern surgery has provided new techniques for bone support that mean a great many more animals are now saved than was once possible.

Horses are put down to save them from the pain, anxiety and shock they suffer with broken bones. This is done when the exact nature of the injury is known. There is no justification for subjecting animals to continued suffering if the end result is not going to allow them a fully useful life. In a high percentage of cases the immediate distress demands immediate relief.

Fractures of small bones like those of the pasterns, sesamoids, knee and hock, are regularly repaired successfully, and animals return sound to normal work. Even bad pelvic fractures with crepitating sounds audible on movement will repair in a high percentage of cases if the affected animal is confined and rested. Some long bone fractures are repaired by surgery involving plating or screwing of bones that lend themselves to this type of therapy (cannon bones being a particular example).

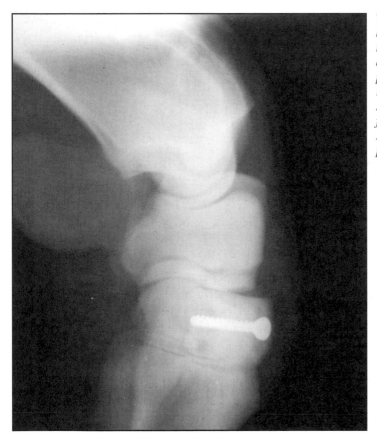

The same bone as pictured on the opposite page; this radiograph shows the fracture with screw in place

However, the strength of materials required to support bones such as the femur and humerus, especially in any animal which will not permit itself to be held in slings, is too great for equipment presently available.

The first principles of bone repair are reduction (bringing the broken bone ends back into apposition) and support. This means that the bone ends should be held in close apposition and immobilised so that healing can take place. Movement is the enemy of fracture repair and may lead to non-union or false joint formation.

Fractures have to be suspected in all acute injuries where there is great pain and the animal is not inclined to put weight on the affected limb. Where there is a clean break in a large bone the diagnosis is easily made, but partial fractures without separation of even the cannon bone will require radiographs to confirm an opinion. In any situation where there is acute pain with a possibility of fracture, even when there is no crepitation on movement of the injured bone or joint, it is always wise to have radiographs taken. Failure to do so can lead to far greater problems later.

However, radiographs are not always successful, especially in picking up cracks or fissures in which there is no bone displacement. The persistence of symptoms may suggest a continuing possibility of fracture and further radiographs should be taken after a week of box rest to try to confirm it.

Scintigraphy is based on the capacity of certain radioactive substances to concentrate in areas of bone injury when injected into a horse. The area is then located by means of a special camera.

Fractures of Individual Bones

Fractures of the scapula, humerus and radius in the forelimb and of the femur and tibia in the hind limb usually mean humane destruction in adult animals, although with foals some cases may be operated on successfully. Fractures of the ulna and fibula are less serious, though ulnar fractures may require surgical treatment to immobilise the broken part with screws. Fracture of any of the carpal bones can be dealt with successfully by surgery.

The pieces of bone from small chip fractures can be removed by arthroscopic surgery and the animal returned to full working soundness in many cases. Slab fractures (larger, block-shaped pieces) can be immobilised by screwing them to the parent bone.

Fractures of the cannon bone are dealt with surgically where there are not too many broken pieces and when there is no serious risk of infection

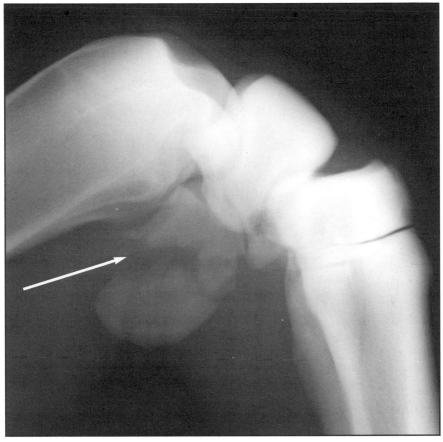

Fracture of the accessory carpal bone

due to contamination when the skin has broken. The health of the tendons and ligaments in the area will also be a consideration. Some fractures can be treated successfully by the use of bone plates and screws to immobilise and support them.

Fractures of a splint bone sometimes heal with rest and support, although in some cases the fractured portion will have to be removed surgically.

Fractures of the proximal sesamoid bones manifest themselves as chips pulled off the extremities or as complete fractures through the substance of the bone. Some of these are surgically treated, the chips being removed and screws used for major fractures. However, many of these would resolve with more conservative treatment.

Fractures of the first phalanx (split pastern) frequently occur in competing animals, and, when there is no displacement, box rest is sufficient

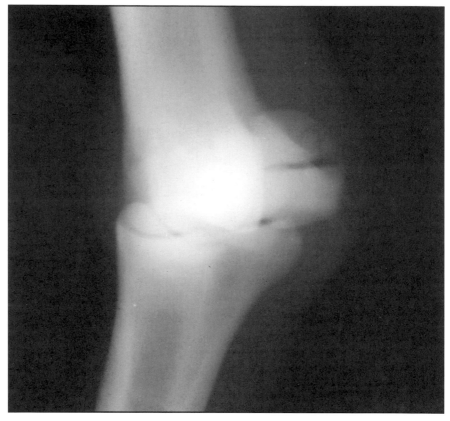

Fracture of the proximal sesamoid bone

to effect a cure in most cases. More complicated fractures may be dealt with surgically or by the application of a cast.

Fractures of the second phalanx are not common while those that occur in the third phalanx frequently heal satisfactorily as long as the coffin joint is not involved.

Fractures of the distal sesamoid (navicular bone) are treated surgically in some cases.

Pelvic fractures, even with fairly severe crepitation, repair successfully if the animal is immobilised. Diagnosis depends on the detection of crepitus and may involve manual rectal examination together with passive limb movement on the affected side. The horse tends to avoid weight bearing on the affected side at rest, and lameness is marked, though not excessive, at the walk.

Fractures of the patella are often the result of a kick and are sometimes successfully treated surgically.

Fractures of the hock, too, are sometimes successfully treated, with immobilisation and rest; however, complicated cases present a poor prognosis. Inevitably, joint disease is a possible complication and each case has to be taken on its own merits.

Fractures of the vertebrae generally offer a poor prognosis, especially if there is any involvement of the spinal cord. Fractures of the spinous or transverse processes may repair without complication if the animal is given rest. Fractures of the sacrum offer a poor prognosis if there is damage to the spinal cord.

Fracture Repair

There is some evidence that bone fracture repair is assisted by magnetic field therapy and electrotherapy, particularly in the absence of infection and if the parts are adequately immobilised. The bones most suited to this form of treatment are those which offer the best prognosis anyway, namely, the smaller bones from the knee and hock downwards. However, if the part is immobilised and supported, the use of this type of therapy assists and quickens healing and prevents the development of non-union fractures.

Ultrasound, contrary to common opinion, is helpful in the treatment of conditions such as pedal osteitis, sesamoiditis and sesamoid fractures without any adverse effect on the bone.

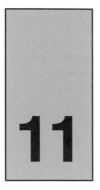

11 Shoeing and Faulty Action

Constant foot care is vital to the wellbeing of all horses, as recognised in the old adage 'No foot - no horse'. This applies particularly to ridden horses and those that work on hard surfaces. It applies equally to the foal and yearling and animals out at grass. Unshod feet in older horses are often brittle and tend to break on dry ground. If the feet of younger horses are correctly balanced it can help prevent the indicidence of developmental diseases, like OCD, and influence the leg conformation these animals will have for the remainder of their active lives.

The purpose of shoeing is to protect the foot from the constant wear caused by hard surfaces, to protect brittle horn from splitting and to diminish the possibility of bruising by removing the sole from close contact with the ground. The aim of shoeing is to provide this protection without disturbing the natural balance of the foot *vis-a-vis* the ground and without disrupting the normal functioning of the foot or its internal structure in any way. In other words, the frog must not be so far removed from the ground that it contracts, and the natural expansion of the heels must not be prevented or concussion absorption and blood circulation will both be inhibited.

The art of shoeing is to make the shoe fit the foot, not the reverse. While this may seem elementary it is not always the case and the practice of making the foot fit the shoe is one that could lead to lameness.

Shoes are applied either hot or cold. Hot shoeing requires a forge, and many farriers carry a portable forge with them. Hot shoeing is preferable to cold shoeing because if the iron is heated it is easier to shape and thus helps to ensure that the shoe is made to fit the foot. With cold shoeing there is always the temptation to make the foot fit the shoe.

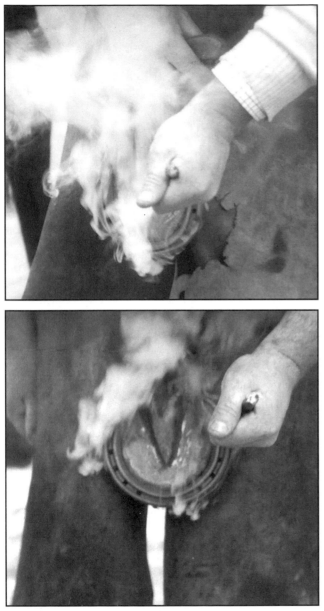

Hot shoeing (left and below)*: the purpose is to make the shoe fit the foot*

Horses are often turned out to grass without shoes. Some tough native breeds have such naturally hard horn that they are never shod, not even when they are ridden. However, the vast majority of ridden horses are shod.

When at grass, horses (particularly Thoroughbreds) may quickly develop broken and cracked hooves, especially if the ground is hard. Their feet may therefore be protected with light tips or half shoes, though there are occasions when owners will decide the feet need a complete rest from the influences of trimming and nailing. Hind shoes are left off to avoid injury from kicking amongst horses turned out together. Whatever the circumstances it is important to check feet regularly and to trim them as needed in order to avoid foot problems when the horse comes back in to work. Foot care should be undertaken on a monthly basis for all horses at grass.

Preparing the Feet of Young Animals

When trimming the feet of foals and yearlings it is essential to keep an eye on the whole limb balance and to trim the feet in a manner that does nothing to disturb this. Problems, such as angular limb deformities, may be caused by simply lifting the foot and trimming it by eye without reference to the rest of the limb. It is therefore vital to examine the limb with the animal in a standing position first and gauge the foot axis with the ground. This must then be related to the whole limb axis and it is important to develop an eye for deviations which may later lead to lameness.

The animal should be walked in a straight line on level ground for a distance of 20m or 30m, so that it is going away from, and back towards, the farrier; the purpose being to see the way in which each limb is protracted and the manner in which the foot meets the ground.

Trimming will vary according to each individual situation and it is therefore not wise to generalise. However, feet that are developing more to the outside than to the inside will need the excess growth removed to bring them back into balance. A foal or yearling with this foot development will tend to move with the toe out, and the foot will wear on the inner side; the whole limb, therefore, will be out of balance and this may place an abnormal strain on the epiphyses of the large metacarpal bone and radius. The strain may be applied to the opposite side of these bones when the opposite occurs and the wear is on the outside of the foot.

In pronounced cases, a threequarter shoe may be needed to control the problem and correct excessive foot wear. Where it is not possible to trim the outer wall back (because of natural wear), but the foot is toeing-out, a threequarter or half shoe placed on the inner side of the foot may be required. This shoe will be made of light iron and reduced in thickness from heel to toe; this is essential because it would not otherwise have the desired effect of balancing the foot. For the opposite problem the shoe would be placed on the outside of the foot.

This kind of shoeing should only be carried out by an experienced farrier who has full knowledge of what is required; it is not a simple cure-all that can be easily understood by the amateur. It is also important to know when the correction has been achieved and when the animal can be returned to normal shoes. Inevitably, it will not be possible to fit iron shoes to very young foals, though plastic may prove of use in some cases.

Preparing the Feet of Adult Animals

The same basic principles apply to preparation of the adult foot. The animal must first be examined while standing flat on level ground and then walked away from and back towards the farrier in all cases. Unfortunately, this simple exercise is not a routine part of shoeing today. The consequence is a great deal of bad shoeing and a high incidence of resulting lameness.

As already stated, the important aspect is that limb balance be considered as a whole and that the foot be trimmed with the express intention of protecting this. Where foot conformation in adult horses is poor and the limb is cast out of balance, correction is required. Failure to appreciate the importance of this is the cause of much lameness today. If, for example, the length of the outer wall exceeds that of the inner wall (encouraging toe-out conformation), the inner wall of the shoe may need to be thicker than the outer to correct this imbalance when it is not possible to correct

Long toe, low at heel, neglected feet with worn shoes

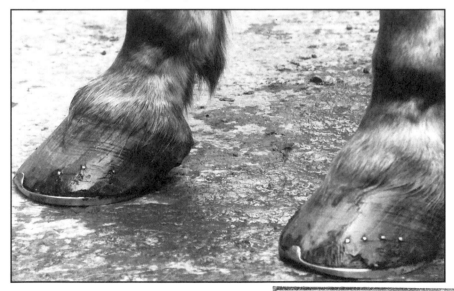

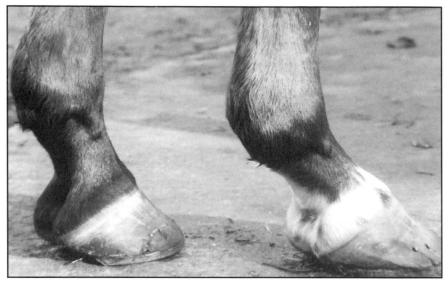

The bulb of the heel is sitting on the right shoe

the defect by trimming. Similarly, if the toe is excessively long and the heel short, it is important to try to restore normal conformation. Heels may need to be raised artificially, or lowered, depending on the situation. This can be done by raising or lowering the natural thickness of the shoes at the heels.

It is critical that, as far as possible, the weight of the horse be trans-

A corrective shoe in place; raising the outside wall in this case

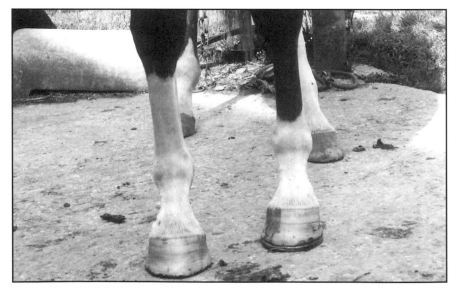

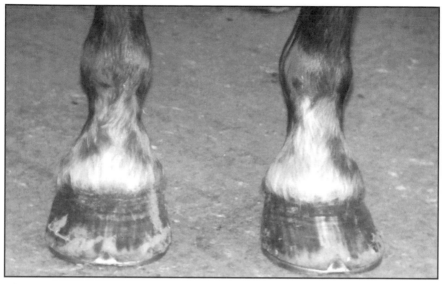

The outer wall of the left fore is splayed out

ferred to the shoe through the wall and bars of the foot only. The shoe must not bear on the sole; when this happens the results are all too clearly seen when the shoe is removed and the foot prepared next time. Bruising beneath the shoe will cause lameness, although the effect may lessen on grass or other soft surfaces. The danger is that an animal feeling its foot and travelling at speed may cause itself even more serious injury by trying to avoid pressure on the affected part.

Shoe Types

The normal shoe fitted for riding horses is an iron shoe, oval in shape with a flat-bearing surface, fullered, and consisting of two branches (divided into heel and quarter) and a toe. Racing plates may be made of light iron or aluminium. Weight is an important factor, and there is no benefit to be had from using iron that is heavier than is absolutely essential. The average shoe is considerably heavier than a racing plate because there is a basic minimum strength required for prolonged normal shoe use which the aluminium shoe does not have.

While replacing shoes regularly is a vital part of foot management, excessive shoeing is a farrier's nightmare. Racehorses are plated for racing and usually have the plates replaced by steel shoes for normal exercise.

Ground surface of a manufactured (machine made) front shoe (Shoe supplied by: Universal Horse Shoes)

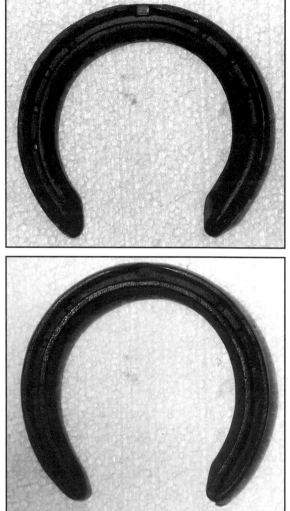

Hand-made front shoe made by the farrier (Shoe supplied by: G. Stonehewer)

With animals which are re-shod constantly the wall of the foot becomes weakened and it is often difficult to find purchase for nails.

Tips

Tip shoes are half-shoes made of light iron which cover the toe and quarter only. They are used for protecting the horn of horses at grass, or for giving height to the toe when the heels need lowering. In the latter case the tip is wedge-shaped from front to rear.

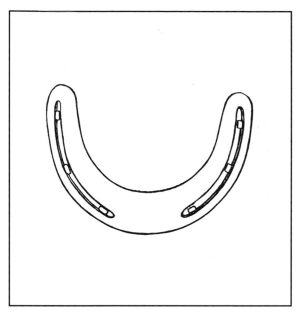

Ground surface of a tip shoe

Threequarter Shoes

One branch of the shoe is shortened in order to avoid pressure on an injured part. This design is also used for yearlings and foals to correct a developing imbalance of the foot. For this purpose either branch may be missing and the shoe is lowered gradually from one end to the other.

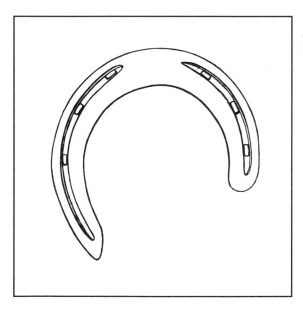

The threequarter shoe is often used to correct foot imbalances

A threequarter shoe in which the bars vary in thickness and the toe is rolled (Shoe supplied by: G Stonehewer)

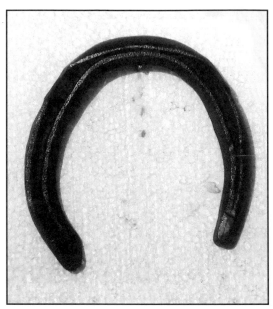

Feathered Shoes

These are used to prevent brushing. The inner branch of the fore or hind shoe is made narrower than the outer branch to prevent striking of the opposite limb. Other efforts to achieve the same end may involve receding the toe or wall, but it is critical in these cases that no contact is made with the sole when the shoe is in place.

Feathered shoe with inner branch narrowed to prevent brushing

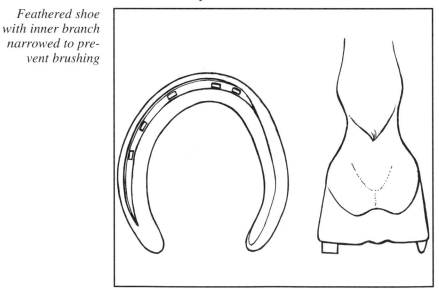

Wedge-heeled Shoes

The heel is raised to relieve pressure on injured tendons, joints or ligaments in convalescent horses. It must be remembered that the recovered
limb will need time to adjust when the shoe is removed. The height to
which a shoe is raised will vary, and may be as much as 4cm to 5cm in
particular cases when an animal is being treated for a condition such as a
sesamoid fracture.

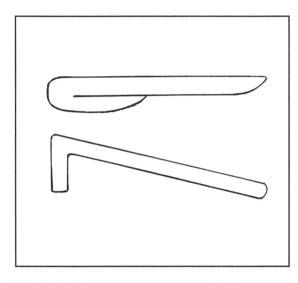

*Wedge-heeled shoes: the
shoe (top) might be used to
raise the heels of a ridden
horse; and (bottom) a shoe
which might be used for
surgical reasons when the
horse is confined*

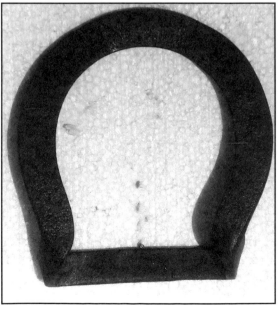

*A type of Patten shoe, used
to raise the heel for
surgical purposes*
(Shoe supplied by: G.
Stonehewer)

Leather Pads for Foot Protection

Feet are fitted with leather pads in order to reduce concussion and protect the sole or frog from bruising. If the sole is flat and the pad is in close contact with it, the use of leather pads is pointless because they simply transfer bruising through to the sensitive sole.

Wedge-shaped Plastic Pads

These are used for sole protection and to give height to the heels where needed. They are often used for horses with long sloping pasterns or low heels to effectively reduce the angle of the foot with the ground. The pads need to be removed regularly because dirt and stones may settle beneath them.

Wedge-shaped plastic pad, ground surface and profile

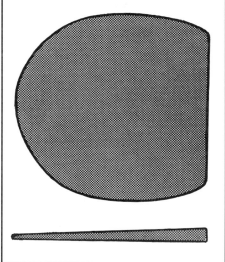

Anti-slipping Devices

Studs are probably the most efficient way to prevent slipping. They are preferred in countries where horses travel on ice and snow. Studs are normally combined with toe-grabs to retain the proper foot axis with the ground.

Studs designed to provide grip on soft surfaces may disturb limb balance if the animal encounters hard ground and may be the cause of joint sprain or other lameness in that case.

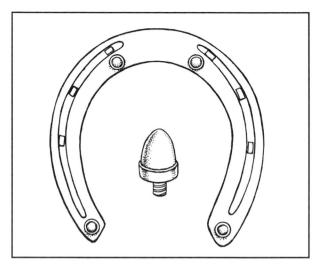

A shoe to which removable studs can be screwed, to prevent horses from losing foothold on slippery surfaces

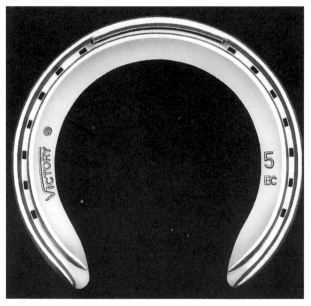

Front aluminium plate, with steel wear inserts (Photo: Victory Racing Company)

Some shoes are made with an anti-slip bearing surface, but they sometimes wear unevenly and the horse is left on a shoe that rocks, leading to possible joint trouble.

Plastic Shoes

Plastic shoes are fitted when there is a problem with normal shoeing, such as that caused by bruising, or inadequate room for nails. The plastic shoes

A racing plate (right); made of a mixture of plastic and aluminium, it can be applied to the horses foot without nails (Photo: Mustad Hoofcare SA)

A modern plastic shoe (below); it is applied to the foot without nails, using glue. The wear is equivalent to that of an average weight steel shoe used under similar conditions (Photo: Mustad Hoofcare SA)

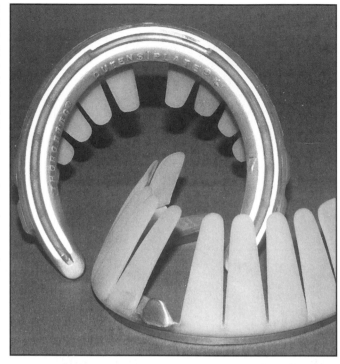

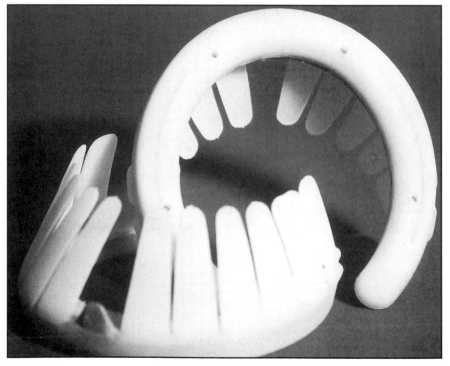

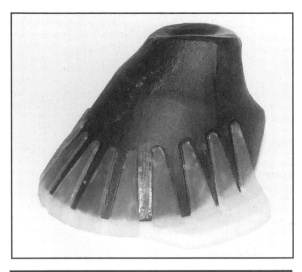

Plastic shoe, as fitted to the foot   (Photo: Mustad Hoofcare SA)

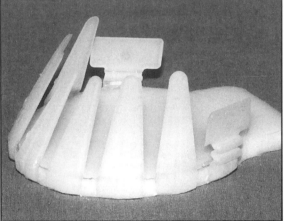

A surgical plastic shoe, particularly useful for shoeing foals   (Photo: Mustad Hoofcare SA)

A lightweight nail-on shoe used to reduce concussion and to which studs can be applied (Photo: Mustad Hoofcare SA)

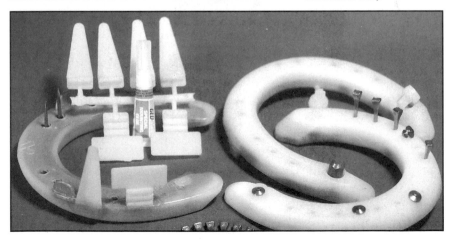

are bonded to the horse's feet and give good wear for about a month. They are a solution to some foot problems in older horses because their design tends to encourage wall support and thus avoid sole contact. Plastic shoes are manufactured in different forms and some have racing plates bonded into them.

A shoe consisting of a wide web aluminium core with shock-absorbing material moulded on to help reduce the effects of concussion (Photo: Victory Racing Company)

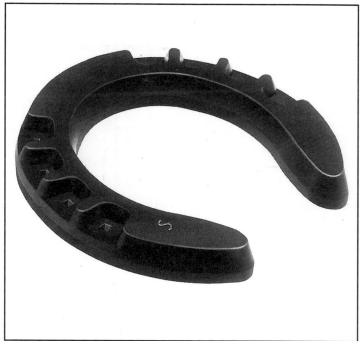

Lightweight wide-web aluminium competition shoe (Photo: Victory Racing Company)

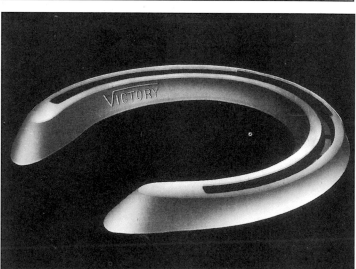

The Heart-bar Shoe

Heart-bar shoes have found a renewed popularity for relieving pain in laminitis. They are made of steel or plastic and their principle purpose is to provide frog support and limit sole contact with the ground. The toe is usually rolled to assist breakover and the heart-bar itself must not extend beyond the limits of the trimmed frog. When fitting the shoe, it is important that the heart-bar comes into contact with the frog before the shoe itself meets the wall.

The heart-bar is too tight if it causes the animal evident discomfort. It must then be readjusted.

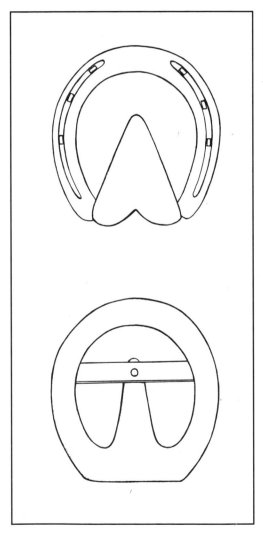

Two heart-bar shoes: an all steel shoe (top), *non-adjustable; and* (bottom) *an adjustable heart-bar shoe which can be all steel or part plastic*

Frog Supports

Frog supports may be purchased from commercial sources or may be made temporarily by use of a rolled cotton bandage placed over the frog and held there by means of elastic adhesive bandage.

The purpose of frog supports, as with the heart-bar shoe, is to provide added foot support and relieve pressure on the painful and inflamed areas of the laminitic foot.

Faulty Action

Horses are said to interfere when they strike a fore or hind limb with the hoof or shoe of the opposite leg. The terms used to describe this relate to the site and type of injury.

Speedy-cutting occurs just beneath the knee and is most often seen in horses with high action. However, the term is not specific and is used for a variety of interferences.

Brushing occurs when a foot (either fore or hind) strikes the opposite foot between the bulb of the heel and the fetlock.

Faulty action: (top row, from left) *speedy cutting, brushing, over-reaching; and* (bottom row, from left) *forging, cross-firing*

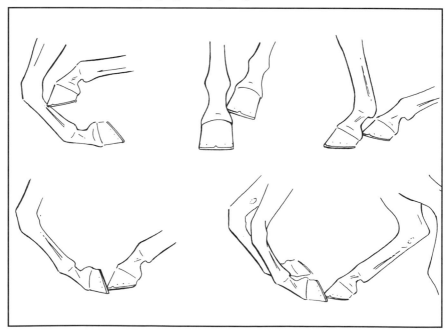

Forging, or clicking, is where the toe of the hind foot strikes the sole of the forefoot on the same, or opposite, side.

Cross-firing occurs when the toe or quarter of the hind foot hits the inside of the forefoot on the opposite side.

A horse is said to 'overreach' when the toe of the hind foot strikes the heel of the forefoot on the same side.

These conditions are most likely to be encountered in young horses shod for the first time, or they may be incurred during the course of a race or other strenuous exercise. They can reflect faulty shoeing or bad action.

The way to prevent them is to first discover the cause and the exact part of the other limb that is responsible for the injury; then the shoeing should be altered in a manner that recedes or removes the offending branch. Protection is also given to the injured region by means of a boot, bandage or other form of barrier.

12 Physiotherapy

The purpose of any form of physical therapy is to promote and foster the natural healing processes of the body. This is done in a number of ways from the simple application of heat and cold, to massage and manipulation and the use of more complex equipment which has the same aim. Heat is applied to dilate blood vessels and encourage blood flow into an area. Applying cold has the opposite effect: it constricts vessels and thus limits the extent of the body's reaction to injury. Heat is applied in the form of poultices to draw infection from wounds. Cold is applied to acute injuries in the form of cold hosing or ice packs to reduce inflammation and control pain, and often provides early relief.

Massage disperses accumulated waste products in muscle (and other soft tissues) and restores normal function to injured areas. As modern horse management does not appear to have room for the time-honoured practice of strapping (the technique of applying a wisp or pad to stimulate muscles) it is noticeable that clinical conditions of muscle have increased considerably.

Whether or not the lack of strapping is a specific cause of the muscle conditions is debatable, but, in any case, the neglect of muscle health will naturally lead to injury problems. There would appear to be a direct correlation here between equine and human athletes (for whom the benefits of muscle massage are known and appreciated).

Manipulation is increasingly used; it has not yet gained the universal approval of the veterinary profession partly owing to a lack of understanding and also to the strong belief that the integrity of the bony spine cannot be disturbed without gross physical symptoms, as might be associated with fracture or dislocation of vertebrae. There is also considerable debate about the mobility of the equine spine segments situated between the cervical and coccygeal areas.

What is being disputed, in fact, is a matter of the degree of mobility. Is it possible to have back pain without vertebral dislocation? The answer, quite simply, is yes, as any human who has suffered back pain will agree. There can be very acute pain associated with very minor movements between spinal structures resulting in possible pressure on nerves and muscle spasm. These symptoms are common in athletic horses, especially those that jump, and the consequences are easily detected by the experienced eye as interferences with normal movement and overt lameness. Manipulation, in a high percentage of cases, brings early relief. Locating the site of origin is a specialised skill, acquired by training, and the relief of symptoms is so commonly achieved as to be beyond criticism. Scepticism is really only a crisis of belief because of the difficulty of explaining the symptoms at a pathological level. Virtually anyone in contact with jumping horses can appreciate the importance of the back in lameness and the success achieved in dealing with it by manipulation.

Therapeutic Ultrasound

Ultra high-frequency sound waves applied with an ultrasound machine can penetrate solid tissue to a depth of as much as 7cm to 10cm (according to different authorities). It is, therefore, beneficial for injuries involving the deep structures of the foot and bones such as the proximal sesamoids. The effect of the sound waves is to promote absorption of fluids, to stimulate circulation of deep parts and assist natural healing. Its effect on bone is, when judiciously used, largely beneficial, and it appears on radiograph that healing is encouraged in fractures of small bones and that re-mineralisation is in evidence in conditions such as pedal osteitis. It is suggested that ultrasound can be dangerous in the region of fractures;

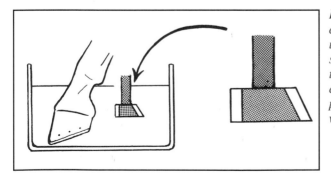

How the lower limb can be treated with ultrasound while submerged in water; the water acting as a coupling medium for passage of the sound waves

however, it appears to be helpful in sesamoid fractures when adequate support and protection are given to the damaged structures. It is also suggested that ultrasound is harmful to sore shins, but neither ultrasound nor laser therapy are curative in this condition; they merely have the effect of reducing pain. The danger then is that more serious injuries will occur as a direct consequence of the loss of pain. When treating bone it is always advised that the machine be worked on a pulsed mode and that the treatment head be constantly moved to avoid undesirable side-effects that may result from the generation of excessive heat. The dosage level should be kept as low as is compatible with successful treatment.

Risks of Ultrasound Use

The following points should be considered.

1)   Where infection is present there is a considerable danger that it may spread to the general system causing septicaemia. Great care must be taken, therefore, to ensure infection is not present before treatment is begun. If there is any doubt, treatment is witheld.

2)   Acute pain may be provoked in the early stages of inflammation and the benefits of using ultrasound in the first day or two after serious injury are doubtful. Slight swellings may be treated earlier. Acute tendon injuries in particular are sensitive to ultrasound therapy at an early stage and may result in manifestations of sharp pain when the treatment head passes over the damaged area.

3)   A coupling agent must be used and the head is moved constantly to prevent overheating of tissues.

4)   When pain is induced the machine should be turned to a pulsed wave mode or the strength reduced or both. Pain is most likely to be noted in the centre of an injury and it is wise to treat only the outer surrounds of an area initially.

5)   Treatment should be limited to a period of not longer than five minutes, though this may be done twice daily in some cases.

6)   Ultrasound is of questionable help where there is haemorrhage, and can even be counter-productive by stimulating fresh bleeding.

7)   By removing the products of inflammation, ultrasound relieves pain and reduces heat. However, it should be appreciated that this may leave an injured area at risk (e.g. tendons may appear to be perfect after treatment but will break down again if not rested until repair is complete). The same may apply to damaged joints and other structures (this effect can be more marked with lasers). Decisions on such matters are best made by experienced people who are qualified to do so. Removing the symp-

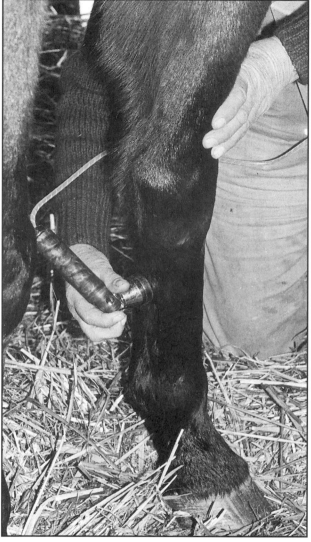

Ultrasonic treatment of the tendon area (Photo: Stuart Newsham)

toms of inflammation can have its advantages but it also can expose an animal to further injury if the dangers are not properly understood.

8)   Ultrasound must not be used in the region of the eyes, brain or reproductive organs.

9)   Heating of the treatment head can mean there is poor coupling and the sound waves are being blocked at the treatment surface. It can lead to crystal damage in the treatment head.

10)   The duration of treatment and strength (measured in watts per square centimetre) are variable with the severity of the condition and are

gauged by operators on the basis of research, experience, and manufacturer's guidelines.

Uses of Ultrasound

1)   For any strain to a joint or its supporting ligaments.
2)   As an adjunct to Faradic-type therapy on damaged muscles.
3)   On tendons and ligaments to reduce inflammation. The limitations of therapy must be appreciated and the structure given adequate time to recover afterwards.
4)   On non-infectious soft swellings (e.g. bursitis).
5)   As an aid to the repair of small-bone fractures (e.g. sesamoids). To relieve the lameness in pedal osteitis.
6)   Treatment of wounds, especially slow-healing wounds.
7)   Control of proud flesh.
8)   Physical injuries to the coronary band respond very well to this type of therapy.

Laser Therapy

Low power, infrared, laser therapy is used for very similar conditions to those treated by ultrasound. It is more effective in its ability to reduce inflammation in certain situations, thereby increasing the danger of animals being returned to work too early. Clinically, there is a marked effect in the reduction of pain, which is possibly why laser therapy is favoured in the treatment of sore shins in young racehorses. However, it must be reiterated that pain relief may lead to the use of lame animals before they are truly sound and that this may have serious consequences.

Neither lasers nor ultrasound will return a chronically damaged muscle to full working use on their own. They will reduce pain and permit treated animals to be worked or raced. However, it is unlikely that the cure will be permanent without artificial muscle contraction returning functional normality to the damaged area.

Faradic Therapy

Faradic therapy (and other forms of electrical muscle stimulation) is widely available today. There is a variety of machines available based on the Faradic principle of intermittent current causing muscle contraction.

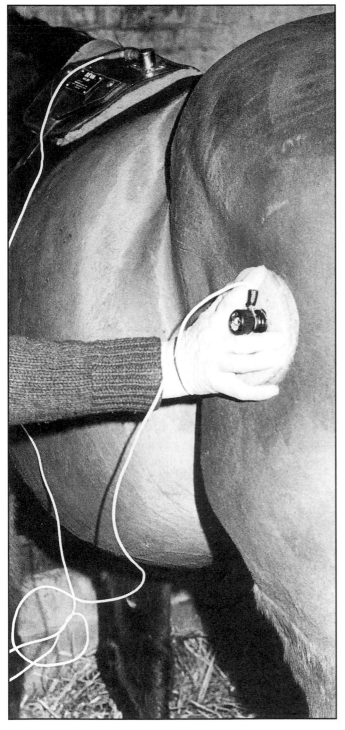

Faradic treatment of the large muscle mass at the front of the thigh (Photo: Stuart Newsham)

Injured muscle does not normally return to use unless stimulated. Other muscle groups take over the function of the injured areas so it may appear that it is being used; this is not so, however, and the consequence is usually minor changes in limb action and dynamics which may well lead to secondary lameness in remote parts.

Faradic stimulation is used as a diagnostic aid, moving the treatment head over whole muscle areas to locate pain and swelling associated with injury. In experienced hands, this is extremely effective. Further treatment of these areas will then, when combined with correct exercise regimes, bring about full recovery. This type of therapy has a vital place in modern horse medicine. It is achieved with the aid of two electrodes (a fixed pad and a moving head in some cases). The pad is placed in contact with the back of the patient and the treatment head is moved over the muscles being examined to stimulate contraction and locate injuries.

A suitable coupling medium must be used to allow contact. Other types of machine working on the same principle use two or more pads which are positioned at either end of the injured muscle.

The machine may operate on a single pole principle with the current applied in one direction. The more modern equipment allows for a bipolar facility with the direction being interchangeable. This permits a different therapeutic effect which is particularly beneficial for soft swellings and joint injuries.

While these machines are available for lay purchase it is important that the standard of application be such that there is no risk to the health of animals. For this reason, it is vital that equine physiotherapy should become a regulated subject with appropriate training courses for those who wish to practice it.

Pulsing Electromagnetic Fields

Although this equipment works on a different basis from lasers and ultrasound its use is aimed at much the same range of conditions. Different pads are supplied with the equipment to enable treatment of various parts of the body.

The equipment works on the basis of magnetic induction, and the current created is repeatedly turned on and off (pulsed), which ultimately means that limited, controlled energy is transferred to the tissue of the animal being treated, and is therefore very safe.

Large pads for back treatment are available and these can be left in place on the animal for extended periods with safety, as can the leg boots.

This form of therapy is considered to have beneficial effects on bone repair.

Magnets

These are used to stimulate circulation in injured areas. They are available incorporated into special boots for various parts of the limbs. Small magnets are also attached to the hoofs with some success in chronic foot conditions.

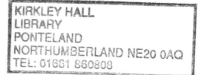

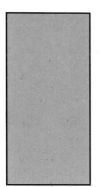

Index

Allen Veterinary Handbooks
LAMENESS

Lameness is a subject of vital importance to every horse owner. Its diagnosis and treatment may be the province of qualified veterinarians, but any horseman will benefit from a deeper understanding of the causes, effects, treatment and prevention.

Peter Gray's book provides explanations for all commonly recognised lameness conditions and challenges the commonly held view that most lameness occurs below the knee. Whilst in no way denying lower limb lameness, the author has found that, when dealing with horses that race, jump or compete in any form of competitive sport, the muscular and skeletal systems are just as often involved.

All relevant aspects of lameness are considered in this book which is essential reading not only for horse owners but also for students and the veterinary profession.

Peter Gray MVB MRCVS trained at University College Dublin and has been in practice since 1964 specialising in thoroughbreds, competition horses and breeding stock. His first book, *Soundness In The Horse* is already regarded as a classic work and his writing is typified both by his deep knowledge and the genuine concern he has for the subject.

Cover illustration by Jacqueline Darnell
Cover design by Nancy Lawrence

Price £13.95

A catalogue of books on horses can be obtained from

J. A. Allen & Co. Ltd.
1 Lower Grosvenor Place,
Buckingham Palace Road,
London, SW1W 0EL

J. A. ALLEN

ISBN 0-85131-577-1

9 780851 315775 >